Library
Knowledge Spa
Royal Cornwall Hospital
Truro
TR1 3HD

01872 256444

This item is to be returned on or before the last date stamped below. To renew items please contact the library Or renew online with your library card number at
www.swims.nhs.uk

21 DAY LOAN

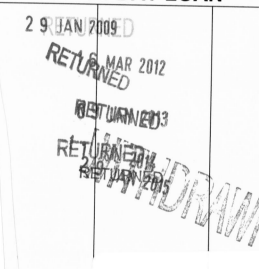
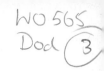

O A L
OXFORD ANAESTHESIA LIBRARY

Anaesthesia for the Elderly Patient

Prof. Chris Dodds

Consultant Anaesthetist,
Department of Anaesthesia,
James Cook University Hospital,
Middlesbrough, UK

Prof. Chandra M. Kumar

Consultant Anaesthetist,
Department of Anaesthesia,
James Cook University Hospital,
Middlesbrough, UK

Dr Frédérique Servin

Service d'Anesthésié et de Réanimation
Chirurgicale, Hôpital Bichat, APHP Paris, France

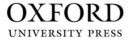

OXFORD
UNIVERSITY PRESS

OXFORD
UNIVERSITY PRESS

Great Clarendon Street, Oxford OX2 6DP

Oxford University Press is a department of the University of Oxford.
It furthers the University's objective of excellence in research, scholarship,
and education by publishing worldwide in

Oxford New York

Auckland Cape Town Dar es Salaam Hong Kong Karachi
Kuala Lumpur Madrid Melbourne Mexico City Nairobi
New Delhi Shanghai Taipei Toronto

With offices in

Argentina Austria Brazil Chile Czech Republic France Greece
Guatemala Hungary Italy Japan Poland Portugal Singapore
South Korea Switzerland Thailand Turkey Ukraine Vietnam

Oxford is a registered trade mark of Oxford University Press
in the UK and in certain other countries

Published in the United States
by Oxford University Press Inc., New York

British Library Cataloguing in Publication Data
Data available

Library of Congress Cataloging in Publication Data
Data available

Typeset by Newgen Imaging Systems (P) Ltd. Chennai, India
Printed in Italy
on acid-free paper by
LegoPrint S.p.A.

ISBN 978–0–19–923462–2

10 9 8 7 6 5 4 3 2 1

Contents

Preface *vii*

Preface

There are more people over 65 years of age than under 16 for the first time in recorded history. Associated with this is an increased longevity resulting in more people than ever reaching their ninth decade or more. These people are much more likely to need access to the highest quality healthcare. Unfortunately, they also suffer the highest rate of complications including death. In some, this is part of an end-of-life process but for others this precipitates them into many years of dependence on others including admission into nursing care despite full independence before becoming ill.

These challenges that they pose to anaesthetists and intensivists are greater than for any other group of patients and yet the entire field remains one of the most poorly researched aspects of medical care.

The aim of this handbook is to provide rapid access to information that will help clinical staff understand some of the problems that occur in caring for the elderly patient. Basic physiological changes and the pharmacological variations with ageing inform the later chapters on the common areas where elderly patients are most likely to present. There are chapters dealing with the commonly occurring presentations of elderly patients, such as emergency surgery and elective orthopaedic, urological, abdominal and neurological surgery.

A brief review of ethics and current law relating to the elderly and anaesthesia has been included to help with understanding the issues of capacity and consent, both of which are areas where the elderly are more likely to require careful assessment and management.

It is hoped that this handbook will not only provide this information in an accessible format but will encourage readers to seek more information on the care of elderly patients, and indeed research into their needs so that we can improve the delivery of effective care for them.

Chris Dodds

Chapter 1

Definitions, social trends and epidemiology

Key points

- The proportion of the elderly is increasing.
- There are now more people over the age of 65 than under the age of 16.
- Dependency increases with advanced age.
- The social and financial costs of dependency are staggeringly large.
- Many countries, medically, spend far more on those over 65 than on those who are younger.
- Elderly cohorts differ markedly – research has a 'sell-by' date.
- Social changes, such as independent living, have a major influence of health care provision.
- Life expectancy is increasing.
- Technological advances will play a major part in the delivery of care to the elderly.
- Anaesthesia still has an important role in maintaining independence.

1.1 Social influences

Changes in population demography are relatively uniform across the world, but these are for differing reasons. Demographic studies show a proportionate increase in the number of the elderly and a decline in numbers of the younger members of society. This may be due to either survival and a falling birth rate in the so-called developed countries or a loss of young adults from infectious disease in other countries. This has a great impact on the finances available to support the health care requirements of an ageing population (Figure 1.1).

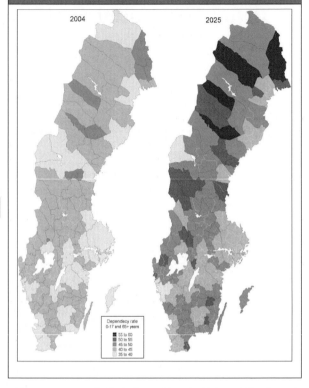

Figure 1.1 Dependency rate 2004 and 2005 per Labour market area (LA)

The proportion of elderly (over 60) and old (over 80) will nearly double over the next 40 years (Tables 1.2 and 1.3). Migration is a further social influence. The elderly may move to rural areas for retirement just as younger people leave for urban areas. At a local level, this may lead to great instability in the ability to fund all the infrastructure necessary to maintain that population: roads, emergency services and hospitals for instance.

Independent living (Table 1.2), causes difficulties for those who may need to be cared for after injury or illness. Several generations may be affected as older parents require care at the same time as

Figure 1.1 is reproduced from Amcoff, J., and Westholm, E. (2007). Understanding rural change – demography as a key to the future. *Futures*. **39**(4): 363–79, with permission from Elsevier.

Table 1.1 Percentage of elderly people co-resident with a child mid to late 1980s/early 1990s

Co-resident (%)	Country
5–15	Denmark, Sweden, Netherlands, Norway, Britain, USA
15–25	France
26–35	Poland, Spain, Hungary
36–45	Italy, Greece
65	Japan

Reproduced with permission from 'Population ageing challenges for policies and programs in developed and developing countries', United Nations Population Fund (1999).

Table 1.2 Percentage of total population aged 60 and over in 1999 and projections for 2050

	1999	2050
World total	10	22
More developed regions	19	33
Less developed regions	8	21
Least developed regions	5	12
Example of regions		
Europe	20	35
Western Europe	21	34
USA	16	28
South America	8	22

Reprinted from *Mechanisms of ageing and development*, Tinker A, 'The social implications of an ageing population', 729–735, (2002), with permission from Elsevier.

do children (Table 1.1). Loss of earnings may be inevitable as more dependency outstrips the local provision of free home-based care, further limiting care options. For many families the cost of nursing care far exceeds the state provided funding (Tables 1.2 and 1.3).

The properties of the 'elderly' also change from one cohort to the next because of differences in nutrition or exposure to infection for instance. These differences make direct extrapolation of data from one group to the next difficult. There is effectively a 'sell-by' date on these studies.

What information is available on the impact of major surgery in the patient population suggests that they have a less favourable outcome and have more complications than younger groups. Recovery is also prolonged and may not allow a return to their previous level of activity. Dependency increases with age and it is estimated that more than 60% of the elderly will be dependent during their last year of life. The cost to carers in the UK is estimated to be £36 billion/year in direct and indirect costs.

Table 1.3 Percentage of population aged 80 and over as a percentage of all aged 60 and over in 1999 and projections for 2050		
	1999	2050
World total	11	19
More developed regions	16	27
Less developed regions	9	17
Least developed regions	7	10
Example of regions		
Europe	15	26
Western Europe	17	31
USA	20	28
South America	11	18

Many of the interventions necessary during surgery, anaesthesia and intensive care that are apparently well tolerated by younger patients cause significant problems in the elderly. These range from the minor (communication difficulties in terminology) to the major (cognitive impairment or loss of independence).

Progressive variation in the pathophysiological make-up of patients is associated with getting older (see Chapter 2). They become more and more individualized in their responses to challenges. This means that the delivery of a standard pattern of care often has unpredictable results.

Legislation, in the form of the Mental Capacity Act 2005, defines new mechanisms for dealing with informed consent and legal capacity in patients with impaired cognition. The full impact of these measures is as yet unclear although there is much useful information on their website (http://www.dca.gov.uk/capacity/index.htm). The predicted increase in numbers of patients with Alzheimer's disease to 840,000 by 2010 means that we will face this problem more frequently, especially in acute situations.

1.2 Recent advances

Basic science research into the causes of ageing are leading some exponents to the belief that longevity could be increased to over 1000 years – a race of 'immortals' being developed as we identify genetic influences involved in malignancy, predisposition to disease and ageing itself. We do not appear to have reached that stage yet but it is clearly a possibility (Figure 1.2).

Table 1.3 is reproduced from Tinker, A. (2002). *Mechanisms of ageing and development:* 'The social implications of an ageing population'. pp.729–35, with permission from Elsevier.

4

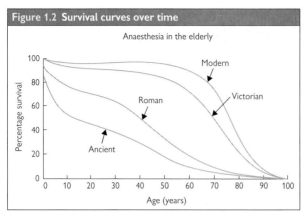

Figure 1.2 Survival curves over time

Anaesthesia in the elderly

More mundane issues include the problem that pre-operative assessment at some time distant from surgery has become established but has problems with detecting acute changes in the elderly and provides only a limited ability to improve the condition of the patient if a problem is detected. Specific testing protocols for major surgery using markers of performance, such as the move of cardiopulmonary exercise testing from being a largely cardiology-based investigation into anaesthetic screening, are showing some promise in risk stratification and the benefits of graded exercise programmes.

At another level, the growing understanding that the impact of injury has on astrocytes is starting to illuminate the possible processes that may lead to the devastating but unpredictable post-operative cognitive dysfunction. At the same time there is also a debate developing on whether volatile or intravenous anaesthetic agents provide benefits or pose risks to patients.

Clinically there have been advances in our understanding of peri-operative management that may make for better outcomes in the elderly. Tight glycaemic control during the peri-operative period for instance does improve outcomes and reduces complication rates post-operatively.

1.3 Novel procedures

The improvement in the success rates of experimental surgery for stem cell implantation mean that it is likely to be of clinical utility within the next few years. The potential to restore or maintain function in degenerative diseases has huge cost implications for the state and for families. They range from chondrocyte resurfacing in major

Permission to reproduce Figure 1.2 sought from Dr Harold T. Davenport.

joints instead of prosthetic replacement, replacement myocardium to repair damage caused by infarction or stereotactic neurosurgical placement of stem cells into the brain to replace key cell lines such as dopaminergic neurones for Parkinson's disease or cholinergic neurones for dementia.

The ability to maintain independence alone makes these attempts worthwhile. However, given the cost benefit to both the patient and the state, these are not going to be inexpensive procedures.

Interventional radiology has been the fastest growing speciality in medicine and has revolutionized many procedures that were once solely the domain of the surgeon. Interventional cardiology has largely replaced coronary artery bypass surgery as first-line management of coronary arterial stenosis. The same technology could allow direct injection of chemotherapy directly into the arterial supply of tumours rather than the whole patient, thus reducing operative surgery for malignancy.

At the same time, newer drugs are changing the face of disease presentation. Statins have deferred the onset of ischaemic heart disease, but not the process – this will mean an increasingly large number of elderly patients presenting with heart disease as a new problem. This will have an impact on our screening of patients as they will, rightly, say they have no cardiovascular disease, but will have organ-specific disease as well as the normal changes of ageing.

1.4 Risk indices

One of the most common methods that is used to try to quantitate the likelihood of a particular operation being of benefit to a patient, or of assessing the risks (morbidity or death) is a calculation of a 'risk index'. The most common method used to test the discriminating power of an index is the 'receiver operating characteristic' (ROC) curve. This plots true positive predictions (sensitivity) against false-positive predictions (specificity). The nearer to unity the area under the curve is, the better model it is. Values above 0.704 are clinically acceptable while pure chance gives a value of 0.5 (Figure 1.3).

These indices have been developed in many countries and can be used in such areas as intensive care medicine (Apache III), major vascular surgery and even to day case surgery. They all have problems in common. The development of a risk index for one population is rarely so predictive in another group because of genetic and environmental impacts related to each group. Extrapolation of a group data set into individual patient outcome is also of limited value. Even large scale, multivariate indices such as those used in risk stratification for cardiac (euroSCORE) or colorectal carcinoma surgery (CR-POSSUM) are of limited predictive value in absolute terms.

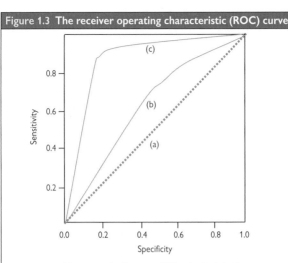

Figure 1.3 The receiver operating characteristic (ROC) curve

(a) = area under the curve of 0.5 and a discrimination
     that is no better than chance;
(b) = small area under the curve and a poor discrimination;
(c) = large area under the curve and a good discrimination.

1.5 **Health care and political issues**

Within each health care system there are limits on the funding available, and the priorities given to that available money. Some of the influences will be related to geographical or social concerns, for instance the need for long distance transfers in remote country areas or the political aspirations of the government. However keeping pace with developments in medical practice across the broad range of specialities is impossible through state provision alone.

One aspect of this is that funding to support clearly identified methods of reducing complications rarely follows immediately, yet the longer it takes for their implementation, the more patients and their carers will suffer avoidable increases in dependency. These range from such simple techniques as active warming or the close control of fluid balance to the provision of an appropriate number of high-dependency beds. This funding inertia alone is likely to actually cost society more than the initial capital investment to deliver these.

Figure 1.3 is reproduced from Adam, S.K. and Osborne, S. (2005). *Critical care nursing – science and practice*, 2nd ed. Figure 17.1, p.513, with permission from Oxford University Press.

There is a drive across the world to increase the proportion of surgery performed as day care or limited stay surgery. This is believed to reduce complications, deliver financial savings and improve patient satisfaction. Initially the scope of surgery offered was limited and often offered to relatively young patients. During the past decade there has been an increase in the complexity of surgery being performed as a 'day case' and limitations related to age have largely disappeared.

Recently, concerns have started to be raised that day case surgery is not without problems. In particular, poor pain relief and cognitive dysfunction persist after such surgery. It is likely that complications that are related to the extent of surgery and the triggered stress responses will occur regardless of the place of care for that patient. Where these are managed within an acute hospital they will be rapidly treated but if they occur in the community they may be less likely to be rapidly identified and treated. Pain relief after intermediate complexity surgery is rarely well provided, yet this has a major influence on subsequent complications such as chest infections.

The costs of providing health care increases year on year, and all systems operate a rationing system. They vary from an explicit definition of state provision with increasing enhancement of medication, facilities, investigations and the like with (insured or self-funding) increasing private investment in some countries to an arbitrary provision of services dependent on local or national taxation and an entirely separate independent health provision. All variations have the potential to unfairly discriminate against the elderly. Even the market place jargon of health economics, such as 'Quality adjusted life years' (QUALYS), makes detrimental assumptions about the quality of life of older patients, especially given the weighting that longer life expectancy gives.

State funding for all aspects of health care are being challenged by the escalating costs of new procedures and therapeutic agents. Changes in management are nearly always more expensive than those now regarded as less useful. Many countries are committed to maintaining the provision of emergency or acute care but are starting to create shared cost care for more elective procedures such as hip replacements. Whether this is by the introduction of semi-private hospitals providing subsidized care or by directly funded private hospitals varies from country to country.

Where these have been in place for years there is little impact on the elderly, but when these are introduced de novo they cause hardship for the retired population of that country. This is because they (the elderly) will not usually have the financial resources to meet these new demands and are often excluded from subscribing to medical health insurance because of the chronic nature of the conditions leading to such elective surgery.

Another issue in these new systems is that they are often advantageously placed to offer surgery or investigations to the fittest, least complicated groups. They limit provision to the chronically ill or those with complex histories because they do not provide the resources, of an intensive care unit (ITU) for instance, which are necessary for the safe care of those patients. This further disadvantages the state provider because it has to continue to deliver care for the complex patients (usually elderly) without the financial buffer of straightforward cases. The divergence in cost per case is then used against the state system to demonstrate how much more effective the new system is.

It is highly unlikely that routine, straightforward elective surgery will continue to be provided by state funding.

1.6 **Patient changes**

The current cohort of proto-aged, the 'baby-boomers', are much more demanding and better informed than previous generations of elderly patients are. The knowledge base on which medical professionalism has been based for centuries is now available at the click of a mouse button. It is information overload rather than ignorance that is the danger now.

Media coverage of all new developments fuels this process and, combined with the surfeit of information, leads to an unrealistic degree of expectation for care provision. This is further aggravated by the TV medical dramas that show recovery from injuries or medical disasters that in real life are far more commonly lethal.

The combination of these influences will mean that the patient/doctor relationship in the future will have to combine acting as an expert adviser on one hand and an access point to health care that may be only partly state funded for routine care.

Face-to-face consultations may become less common as access to investigations and imaging will be available by direct booking, and the interpretation of these findings may be by experts in other parts of the world. Robot-based medical history taking and diagnostic evaluations are already being used, and it may only be a matter of time before interventional medicine and surgery do not require human delivered physical contact.

1.7 **Summary**

The elderly are vulnerable to the stresses of injury, surgery and anaesthesia, which may profoundly affect their quality of life as well as its length. Understanding the changes in society and the imperatives that an ageing population places on governments is vital if we are to protect and preserve the independence and well-being of our elderly patients.

Further reading

Amcoff J and Westholm E. Understanding rural change – demography as a key to the future. *Futures* 2007; **39**: 363–379.

Hutton P, Cooper GM, James III FM and Butterworth IV JF, Eds. *Fundamental Principles and Practice of Anaesthesia*. Martin Dunitz ltd, UK 2002 IABN 1-899066-57-8. Chapter 43.

Chapter 2

Pathophysiological changes of ageing and their relevance to anaesthesia

Key points

- Organ function declines at an average rate of 1% a year from the age of 40.
- Behavioural influences (choosing not to drink for instance) have to be considered.
- Atrial fibrillation (AF) is the default rhythm for the elderly.
- Closing volume lies within tidal ventilation when supine after the age of 65.
- Muscles are no longer 'vessel-rich'.
- Autonomic dysfunction may be occult but should be sought.
- Renal homeostasis is reduced in both speed and degree of compensation to water and solute loads.

Ageing is a balance between gradual maturation and senescence, which is the process by which the capacity for cell division and the capacity for growth and function are lost over time ultimately leading to death. The changes that occur with ageing can be categorized as those that result from ageing itself and those that result from diseases, lifestyle and exposures. Normal ageing describes the changes attributed to ageing itself, but these are often associated with common complex diseases and functional impairments. However, this complex impairment is hard to define because people age very differently. Some develop disease with impaired organs while others seem to escape disease altogether. 'Healthy ageing' refers to a process by which the deleterious effects are minimized, preserving function until senescence makes continued life impossible. People who age successfully avoid experiencing many of the undesirable effects of ageing and whether they have a disease or not, remain both physically and mentally functional.

Progressive cell loss occurs at a variable rate in individual patients and their organ systems. Functional reserve is the difference between the basal level of organ function at rest and the maximum level of organ function that can be achieved in response to increased demand such as during exercise or in response to surgical stress. Functional reserve is generally reduced in elderly patients leading to increased morbidity and mortality. This decreased functional reserve is difficult to detect. Patients may have limited mobility and as a result are unable to exert themselves. These patients usually are unaware that they could suffer from breathlessness or angina but they may have significant underlying and undetected ischaemic cardiac disease.

2.1 **Organ dysfunction**

Age-related changes occur in all organs (see Figure 2.1) but the reduction is especially pronounced in the cardiovascular, respiratory, renal and central nervous system. It is important to understand these changes as they largely determine the outcome of surgical procedures under both general and regional anaesthesia.

2.2 **Cardiovascular system**

With age, the heart can atrophy, remain unchanged or develop moderate or marked hypertrophy. Atrophy usually coincides with various wasting diseases and is not observed during ageing in healthy persons. The cardiac mass increases by approximately 1–1.5 g every year. There is an age-related modest increase in the left ventricular (LV) wall thickness even in patients free of cardiovascular disease or hypertension. Studies that have excluded subjects with hypertension, however, show consistent increases in LV wall thickness in conjunction with reduced diastolic compliance, and the stimulus for hypertrophy may be an increased after-load imposed on the LV by an age-related decline in aortic compliance. All types of hypertrophy are associated with various degrees of increased deposition of collagen, which may further reduce diastolic compliance. The amount of fibrous tissue within the myocardium increases with age but does not contribute appreciably to cardiac mass.

The valvular structures are affected by ageing that is manifested by thickening of the aortic and mitral leaflets and a gradual increase in the circumference of all four cardiac valves. Frequently the mitral and aortic valves are the sites of ectopic calcification that results from degeneration of the collagen content. Calcification of the mitral apparatus is common in elderly patients particularly in women and

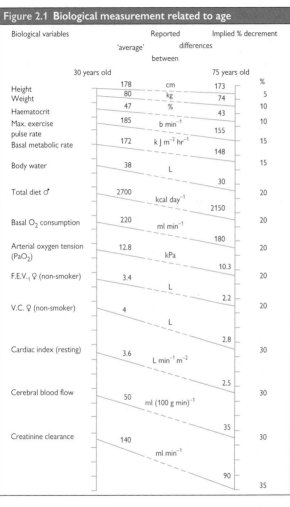

Figure 2.1 Biological measurement related to age

Biological variables		Reported	Implied % decrement
	'average'	differences	
		between	

	30 years old		75 years old	%
Height	178	cm	173	
Weight	80	kg	74	5
Haematocrit	47	%	43	10
Max. exercise pulse rate	185	b min^{-1}	155	10
Basal metabolic rate	172	k J m^{-2} hr^{-1}	148	15
Body water	38	L	30	15
Total diet ♂	2700	kcal day^{-1}	2150	20
Basal O$_2$ consumption	220	ml min^{-1}	180	20
Arterial oxygen tension (PaO$_2$)	12.8	kPa	10.3	20
F.E.V.$_{-1}$ ♀ (non-smoker)	3.4	L	2.2	20
V.C. ♀ (non-smoker)	4	L	2.8	20
Cardiac index (resting)	3.6	L min^{-1} m^{-2}	2.5	30
Cerebral blood flow	50	ml (100 g min)$^{-1}$	35	30
Creatinine clearance	140	ml min^{-1}	90	30
				35

13

patients with systemic hypertension or diabetes mellitus. Mild degrees of mitral regurgitation (MR) are common but clinically significant MR is much less common. A 12-fold increase in the incidence of atrial fibrillation (AF) is seen and conduction defects frequently occur as well. Histological changes detected in the vasculature include increased

Figure 2.1 is reproduced from Davenport, H.T. (1988). *Anaesthesia and the Aged Patient*, with permission from Blackwell Publishing.

intimal thickness, elastin fragmentation and increased collagen content of the arterial wall. The resultant decrease in compliance reduces distensibility and causes a measurable increase in pulsed-wave velocity. In the presence of atherosclerotic disease, these findings are accentuated and may explain the age-related increases in LV wall thickness.

Peak contractile force of the myocardium remains unimpaired in the ageing myocardium but the duration of contraction is prolonged. This may be due to diminished calcium uptake by the myofibrillar sarcoplasmic reticulum. The Frank–Starling length–tension relationship remains unchanged in the senescent heart, although the augmentation of contractility by cardiac glycosides and β-adrenergic stimulation is blunted in the senescent myocardium.

Ischaemic heart disease is common and is caused by smoking, and conditions such as hypercholesterolaemia, hypertension, type 2 diabetes mellitus and obesity contribute to the development of atherosclerosis. This results in a less compliant arterial tree, increased systemic vascular resistance and systemic hypertension leading to LV hypertrophy, reduced ventricular compliance and contractility and eventually reduced cardiac output.

The resting cardiac index (cardiac output per unit of time [L min^{-1}], measured while seated and divided by body surface area [m^2]) is not reduced in healthy older men who have been rigorously screened to exclude occult heart disease and who live independently in the community. However, in older women, resting cardiac output decreases slightly because neither end-diastolic volume nor stroke volume increases to compensate for the modest reduction in heart rate. Stroke volume decreases, systole time is prolonged and, with a decrease in ventricular contractility, cardiac output and its reserve decline. Despite this, the average arterial pressure rises with an increase in the systolic and a slight drop in the diastolic pressures. The mean arterial pressure remains unchanged. Peripheral vascular resistance increases progressively. Progressive coronary arterial sclerosis leads to a reduction in maximal coronary artery blood flow. Vessel walls become less compliant as smooth muscle is reduced and collagen replaces elastin. Major vessels become stretched and distended damaging the endothelium and baro-receptors leading to a labile blood pressure. Importantly, any increase in intrathoracic pressure, passively or actively, causes proportionately greater decreases in blood pressure with little or no rebound elevation. With age, the supine resting heart rate does not change in healthy men; the heart rate while seated decreases slightly in men and women. Spontaneous variations in heart rate during a 24-hour period decrease in men without coronary artery disease, as do variations in the sinus rate with respiration. The intrinsic sinus rate (i.e. measured after sympathetic and parasympathetic blockade) decreases significantly with age. Cardiac output increases by increasing stroke volume rather than increasing heart rate. There is reduction in vasomotor tone; both vagal and sympathetic influences are minimized. Degenerative vasomotor control precipitates syncope in the presence of decreased cardiac output or peripheral resistance. Postural hypotension can be spontaneous or due to an effect of drugs. The reduced cardiac output compromises blood flow to the kidneys and brain. The resting ejection fraction is not reduced in healthy older men and women. Resting stroke volume increases slightly in older men (commensurately with the slightly larger end-diastolic volume) and remains constant in older women. Autoregulation of blood flow to these organs is impaired in the elderly; hence kidneys and brain are more prone to peri-operative ischaemia.

Atrial pacemaker cells decline in number and fall to approximately 10% of its adolescent value by the age of 70. This makes AF the 'default' rhythm for the elderly. Myofibrils enlarge but become less numerous. Collagen and fat replace a substantial volume of the muscle mass. Deposits of amyloid and subendocardial calcification impair conduction in the ventricle. This combined with a reduction in pacemaker cells make the elderly prone to arrhythmias. The fast ventricular rate in AF leads to poor and variable diastolic filling and a reduced cardiac output that is not tolerated well in an elderly patient. If AF is shown to cause haemodynamic instability, cardioversion should be considered before anaesthesia to control heart rate to <100 min^{-1}.

Ageing affects aerobic capacity and cardiovascular performance during exercise. Peak exercise capacity and peak oxygen (O_2) consumption decrease with age, but inter-individual variation is substantial. Aerobic capacity decreases by 50% between the ages of 20 and 80 because maximum cardiac output decreases by 25% and also peripheral O_2 utilization decreases because of age-associated reductions in muscle mass and strength. During all levels of exercise, the older heart, on average, pumps blood from a larger filling volume. However, stroke volume in older persons does not exceed that in younger persons, because the end-systolic volume in older persons remains larger than it does in younger persons. Consequently, the ejection fraction does not increase as much in response to an increase in end-diastolic volume. Thus, although the stroke volume during exercise is maintained at the same level in older persons as in younger persons, the Frank–Starling mechanism is blunted with age. These changes result from a combination of age-associated factors, including augmented vascular and cardiac components of after-load, reduced maximal intrinsic myocardial contractility and reduced augmentation of contractility by β-adrenergic stimulation.

The activity of the sympathetic nervous system seems to increase with age, as suggested by higher blood levels of norepinephrine and epinephrine in older than in younger persons during any effort. Because levels of norepinephrine and epinephrine are higher, more β-adrenergic receptors on cardiac and vascular cell surfaces are occupied. The result is a desensitization of β-adrenergic receptors, thereby causing a down-regulation of associated intracellular signalling pathways.

The physiological response to stress such as hypovolaemia may be blunted due to reduced baro-receptor sensitivity and autonomic function. This may be significant if the patient is also taking β-blockers or angiotensin-converting enzyme (ACE) inhibitors. A normal response to exercise in young patients is increased heart rate and ejection fraction. This response is blunted in elderly patients due to decreased reactivity of β-receptors and the ejection fraction may even fall further. Maximum cardiac output and hence functional cardiac reserve decreases as age increases.

The elderly have reduced haemoglobin and haematocrit as well as reduced marrow iron stores. They can suffer from anaemia following even trivial haemorrhage. However, blood transfusion is not without problems and is considered only once other serious causes of anaemia are excluded or functional limitation is present.

Other haematological changes include reduced cellular immune response because of thymic atrophy and a reduction in the number of T cells. Lymphocytosis within the marrow results in susceptibility to proliferative disorders and infections.

2.3 Respiratory system

Ventilatory responses to hypoxia, hypercarbia and mechanical stress diminish with ageing because peripheral and central chemoreceptor responses diminish, as does the integration of central nervous system pathways. Ageing also decreases neural output to the respiratory muscles and lower chest wall, and this reduces lung mechanical efficiency. These reductions increase the risk of developing hypoxia and hypercapnia if the elderly acquire disorders that decrease oxygen levels. The respiratory adverse effects of benzodiazepines, opioids and volatile anaesthetic agents are exaggerated.

Reduced height and calcification of vertebral column lead to a barrel chest appearance. The diaphragm is flattened, intercostal muscles are weak and the chest wall rigid. These not only increase the work of breathing but also reduce its efficiency. In the presence of a disorder that requires sustained increases in ventilation, it predisposes the elderly to hypoxaemia and hypercapnia, thus possibly the need for mechanical or assisted ventilation. The chest and lung compliances

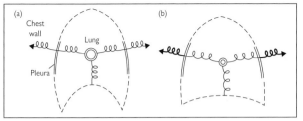

Figure 2.2 Lung volume and elastic recoil in (a) normal healthy volunteer and (b) elderly patient, in the latter showing increased lung volume and reduced elastic recoil resulting in reduced compliance and decreased ventilation

change and chest becomes less compliant. Changes in compliance are primarily responsible for age-related decreases in ventilation and the corresponding decreases in gas distribution that result from the collapse of small airways. Cellular changes also occur in the lung parenchyma. Elastic recoil of the lungs is reduced with altered surfactant production, increasing the lung volume at end-expiration, which in turn increases the residual volume (see Figure 2.2). Airway collapse is prevented by the intra-alveolar pressure generated by the elastic recoil of the lungs. Loss of recoil results in a collapse of poorly supported peripheral airways resulting in decreased flow at low lung volumes. Airway collapse, increasing dependence on the diaphragm and abdominal muscles and reduced vital capacity all produce an uneven distribution of ventilation, without change in tidal volume at rest. The upper airway becomes increasingly unstable during inspiration, and this is most marked during sleep. There is a progressive increase in the number of episodes of airway collapse and arterial oxyhaemoglobin desaturations during sleep with advancing age. Snoring (partial upper airway obstruction) is almost universal. Silent aspiration is common. This is partly due to the fall in sensitivity of the cough reflexes – a seven-fold reduction – and partly due to increased oesophageal reflux with ageing. The increasingly negative intrathoracic pressure necessary to overcome the high resistance of the upper airway further aggravates these problems.

Total lung capacity is relatively unchanged (Figure 2.3). The volume at which small dependent airways start to close (closing capacity) increases with age. Change in the relationship between functional residual capacity and closing capacity causes an increased ventilation perfusion mismatch. There is a parallel decrease in the vital capacity. Widening of the airways together with an increase in the size of the

Figure 2.2 is reproduced from Davenport, H.T. (1988). *Anaesthesia and the Aged patient*, with permission from Blackwell publishing.

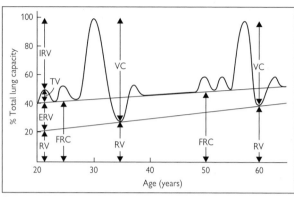

Figure 2.3 Effects of ageing: total lung capacity remains unchanged, closing capacity increases with age, vital capacity decreases with age and residual volume increases

alveolar ducts increases the anatomical dead space. Reduction in elastic fibres in these ducts may explain why airway closure occurs at resting functional residual capacity. This premature closure of the airways further contributes to increases in residual volume. By the mean age of 65, not all the airways are opened during tidal breathing in the sitting position. Atelectasis and potentially a complicating pneumonia are more likely to develop in the elderly, particularly when lying in bed for a prolonged period.

Increases in pulmonary vascular resistance and pulmonary artery pressure occur with age and may be secondary to decreases in cross-sectional area of the pulmonary capillary bed. The alveolar–arterial oxygen tension difference increases causing a gradual decrease in the partial pressure of oxygen in arterial blood (PaO_2). The maximum oxygen consumption describes the body's ability to maximally deliver oxygen to the tissues and this gradually declines with the passing of each decade due to reduction in maximal heart rate, muscle mass and cardiovascular deconditioning associated with lower levels of physical activity or from changes in cardiovascular function. The $PaCO_2$ usually remains unchanged. Diffusing capacity declines gradually with every decade after adulthood due to decreased alveolar-capillary surface area caused by inflammation-induced destruction of capillary containing alveolar walls. The loss of alveolar-capillary surface area decreases venous oxygenation, particularly under condition of high pulmonary blood flow (see Figure 2.4). Fibrous replacement of the muscular arterial media and reduction in the number of capillaries increases the pulmonary vascular resistance and shunting.

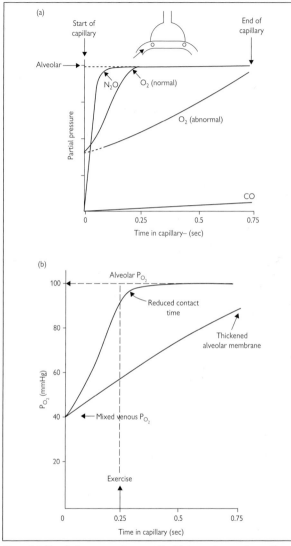

Figure 2.4 The effect on oxygenation caused by (a) changes in anaemia or with abnormal haemoglobins and (b) effects of diffusion and capillary transit time

Figure 2.4 is reproduced with permission from Berne, P.M. *et al. Physiology*, 5th ed, p.500, Elsevier.

Maximal pulmonary blood flow, and therefore perfusion, is lowered. The additional oxygen demand caused by increased activity induces increased ventilation in the presence of a diminished maximum breathing capacity. This leads to dyspnoea in the absence of underlying pulmonary disease.

Any alteration in the control of respiration, lung structure, mechanics and pulmonary blood flow predispose elderly patients to peri-operative complications. Atelectasis, pulmonary embolism and chest infections are all more common in elderly patients, particularly following abdominal or thoracic surgery. Progressive weakness of intercostal and accessory muscles reduces the ability to cough forcibly. The rate of mucociliary transport declines with ageing. The bronchial mucosa degenerate because of impaired blood supply and the cilia are ineffective in keeping the small airways clear, particularly in smokers. Cellular immunity declines with age. Dysphagia and other swallowing difficulties and impaired oesophageal motility occur more often in the elderly and increase the risk of aspiration and chest infection. Early mobilization and good analgesia following abdominal surgery help reduce lung atelectasis and collapse.

2.4 **Renal function**

Renal function does not deteriorate in everyone with age; in some it remains relatively unchanged, in others it deteriorates only slightly and in still others there is a more substantial decline. Pragmatically, renal function must be considered to be reduced in elderly patients who are admitted as an emergency.

Renal mass may decrease as much as 30% by the age of 80. Loss of mass is most prominent in the renal cortex and co-relates with a decreased number of functioning glomeruli. There is a failure of the countercurrent gradients in the loop of Henle. Ageing also affects the collecting system, and prostate disease in men and urinary incontinence in women will have complex effects on the behaviour of the patient. Active, self-imposed fluid restriction is quite common as an attempt to limit the impact of these conditions, especially if bed-bound in an acute hospital environment.

Renal blood flow decreases about 10% per decade due to a decrease in the reno-vascular bed. Cortical blood flow decreases but medullary flow is preserved. Vascular changes may initiate this deterioration. As renal blood flow is reduced, glomerular filtration and concentrating ability decline linearly at about 1% per annum from 30 to 80 years. The decrease in glomerular filtration rate is measured by creatinine clearance. Glomerular filtration rate and creatinine clearance decrease with age but the serum creatinine remains relatively unchanged. This is because muscle bulk also decreases with age resulting in reduced creatinine production. Therefore, serum creatinine level is a poor predictor of renal function in the elderly. Large acid or alkali loads can overwhelm the ability of the kidney to maintain acid–base homeostasis.

Tubular function is also impaired with reduced renal concentrating ability and reduced free water clearance. Diverticula appear in the distal nephron, reaching a peak of about three per tubule by age 90. These diverticula may become retention cysts. Clearance of renally excreted drugs is reduced, and fluid balance is more critical as responses to both fluid loading and dehydration are impaired. Renal function may deteriorate rapidly in hypovolaemic patients, particularly those taking non-steroidal anti-inflammatory drugs (NSAIDs) or ACE inhibitors. Close monitoring of hourly urine output after major surgery should be routine.

2.5 **Fluid and electrolyte balance**

Renal capacity to conserve sodium is decreased. With ageing there is nephron loss and a consequent increase in the osmotic load per nephron. Renin levels are decreased in both basal and stimulated states. As a result of the changes in renin, aldosterone levels are decreased. This age-related decrease in renin and aldosterone levels contributes to the development of various fluid and electrolyte abnormalities. Elderly patients have tendency to lose sodium because of poor dietary habits. There is a decrease in angiotensin II production, which results from lack of renin stimulation, and this leads to the impairment of tubular concentrating ability. There is a decreased thirst response. Inadequate salt intake and impaired thirst response lead to dehydration and sodium depletion. Generally there is no change in serum sodium, potassium, hydrogen ion concentration or circulating blood volume with age but adaptive mechanisms may be impaired. Therefore, acute illness is often complicated by derangements in fluid and electrolytes balance.

Elderly patients with or without cardiovascular disease are at increased risk from rapid volume expansion. They are less able to excrete an elevated salt load requiring a longer time to re-establish balance. These changes may be due to decreased glomerular filtration rate and decreased baro-receptor reflex sensitivity. Potassium handling and renal excretion of potassium is altered with age. The tendency towards hyperkalaemia is enhanced by acidosis because the ageing kidney is slow to correct an increase in acid load, resulting in prolonged depression of serum pH and a shift of potassium out of cells. All these factors lead to increased serum potassium. Dehydration with altered electrolytes is common when fluid intake is limited and insensible loss is increased.

2.6 **Nervous system**

In the absence of neurological disease, intellectual performance tends to be unchanged until at least the age of 80, but tasks may take longer to perform. Verbal skills are well maintained until the age of 70, after which some healthy elderly gradually develop a reduction in vocabulary and tend to make semantic errors. The elderly with neurological disease are especially susceptible to the action of many anaesthetic drugs.

An age-related decline in central nervous system function is common. The causes of this decline include cerebrovascular disease, changes in hormone levels, neuronal damage induced by oxidative stress as well as a generalized progressive loss of cells. Brain weight declines about 10% and the area of the cerebral ventricles relative to the entire brain may decrease three to four times. Plasticity at the nerve cell level involves compensatory lengthening and production of dendrites in remaining nerve cells to offset the age-related gradual deterioration and loss of nerve cells. New connections in the dendritic tree may compensate for the fewer nerve cells. Other compensatory changes occur when the brain is damaged (the non-dominant hemisphere may compensate when speech centres in the dominant hemisphere are damaged leading to gradual improvement in speech function). Other motor systems may compensate when large areas of cerebellum are destroyed by injury, vascular disease or tumour. Compensatory mechanisms are more effective in higher centres. The ability to compensate after any damage in spinal cord declines with age.

Confusion is more common, both pre- and post-operatively. Cognitive impairment increases with ageing, and dementia may affect up to 20% of patients over the age of 80. Dementia should be diagnosed only by formal testing, and ideally by experts in geriatric psychology. It is not a diagnosis to be made lightly because it has a 50% life expectancy of fewer than 5 years – similar to most malignant carcinomas. Attention span falls, factual recall becomes impaired and repeated explanations are necessary. Mental impairment is present in up to 5% of the population and is associated with illiteracy. Changes in cognitive function are multifactorial. Of the octogenarians, 20% have some degree of dementia, but this diagnosis should be made only when other causes have been excluded. Causes of dementia include hypoxia, infection, drug toxicity, electrolyte abnormalities, hypoperfusion, hypotension, hypothyroidism, constipation and impaired sight or hearing.

Autonomic dysfunction is prevalent in the ageing population and may result in labile blood pressure and peri-operative arrhythmias. The baro-receptor reflex may be attenuated leading to postural hypotension and a decrease in blood pressure during anaesthesia particularly during induction of anaesthesia especially if hypovolaemic. Impaired temperature regulation and delayed gastric emptying may also occur. A rapid sequence induction is desirable in such cases.

Temperature regulation is impaired in the ageing population and there is a poor physiological compensatory mechanism such as shivering. Hunger and thirst centres are down-regulated and antidiuretic hormone is less effective making the elderly vulnerable to dehydration and malnutrition. The peripheral nervous system declines in a similar manner. Nerve conduction velocity decreases, and appreciation of pain reduces. The elderly generally do not complain about pain although they suffer as much as younger patients.

Cerebral blood supply is reduced by 20% on an average as a result of atheroma or sclerosis. Vertebrobasilar insufficiency is not uncommon. Decreases are greater in certain areas of the brain (pre-frontal area) and are greater in the grey matter than in the white matter. Flexion or extension of the neck can compromise cerebral oxygen delivery. Osteoporosis and laxity of ligaments is common in old age and care should be exercised during induction of anaesthesia.

Free radicals (atoms or molecules with unpaired electron) that are produced normally during metabolism accumulate with age and may have a toxic effect on nerve cells. With a generalized progressive loss of cells, there are losses of neurotransmitter systems such as active nuclei of the cholinergic and dopaminergic systems. Cholinergic receptors and catecholamine levels usually decrease. The loss in function that this causes is masked by the degree of reserve that exists; it is estimated that a loss of 70–80% of dopaminergic function is necessary before symptoms are seen in patients with Parkinson's disease. There is an increase in monoamine oxidase levels. When this increase is inhibited by monoamine oxidase inhibitors, the onset of disability in patients with Parkinson's disease may be forestalled. The apoptosis that occurs in neuronal cells with ageing may be exacerbated by stress responses, especially the rises in cortisol.

2.7 Hepatic system

Liver mass decreases with age. Hepatic blood flow decreases by 10% per decade. There is a decreased capacity to metabolize drugs. This decreased metabolic activity and reduced hepatic blood flow alters the pharmacokinetic and pharmacodynamics of many drugs used during anaesthesia (see Chapter 3).

2.8 Endocrine system

The ageing process is associated with glucose intolerance. This intolerance is due to many factors, including insulin resistance, dysregulation of insulin secretion, alterations in insulin receptor number or post-receptor defects. The incidence of diabetes is increased in the elderly, and may be seen in up to 25% of patients aged over 80 years. Diabetics frequently have cardiovascular, renal, neurological and visual impairment and require control of blood glucose levels during the peri-operative period. The metabolic clearance rate of thyroid hormone decreases with age. With an intact hypothalamic–pituitary thyroid axis, thyroxine levels are maintained in the normal range. Yet, with thyroid disease, when exogenous thyroxine is administered, the replacement dose must be reduced to account for the change in clearance. There is a decreased oesterogen production, a notable alteration in bone metabolism and increased incidence of osteoporosis.

2.9 **Nutrition**

Malnutrition is common in the elderly and is associated with increased morbidity and mortality. Nutritional supplementation is generally advocated to reduce the length of hospital stay and post-operative complications. Oral protein supplementation is advised in those with significant malnutrition.

2.10 **Musculoskeletal system**

Arthritis is almost universal in the elderly, and this will limit their ability to exercise.

Degenerative diseases of all types affect the elderly. This may limit exercise tolerance; hence it is difficult to assess fitness. This may mask a falling exercise tolerance due to cardiorespiratory failure. It also leads to severe pain post-operatively if there has been an excessive manipulation under anaesthesia. Osteoporosis and ligament laxity make epidural and spinal anaesthesia technically difficult. These patients are prone to fractures or dislocation of joints (including the cervical spine) while anaesthetised. Care should be taken with patient movement and intra-operative positioning as vigorous movements of the patient or pressure over joints may lead to fracture or dislocation. Vulnerable pressure points should be well padded.

2.11 **Vision**

Visual acuity may decrease because of changes in the retina or neural element. Blindness affects nearly 30% of the elderly, largely due to cataracts and glaucoma, and may make understanding written material such as consent forms and visual analogue pain scales very difficult. Diminished tear production and secretion lead to dry eyes, thus predisposing corneal damage.

2.12 **Hearing**

Deafness is more common and may be severe in about 35% of elderly patients. There are changes in both the peripheral and central auditory systems in elderly patients. A loss of hearing pure tones, especially in higher frequencies, is more pronounced and can interfere with both hearing and understanding speech. Brain stem changes may lead to difficulty in hearing and localising sounds in noisy environments. Cortical changes may lead to problems with difficult speech and language.

An increasing elderly population and advances in surgical technology present many challenges to anaesthetists. Many elderly patients are likely to undergo surgery. Increased age and pre-existing illness both increase the incidence of complications. Signs and symptoms are often masked by limitation of movement and lack of exercise because of the pain of arthritis. A successful outcome depends on meticulous attention to pre-operative assessment and an intelligent choice of suitable anaesthetic techniques. Therefore, the opportunity to improve physiological function pre-operatively, where applicable, should never be missed. To provide safe and effective anaesthesia, an understanding of the limitations of physiological function in the elderly is of paramount importance.

Further reading

Chelluri L. Critical Illness in the elderly: Review of pathophysiology of aging and outcome of intensive care. *J Intensive Care Med* 2001; **16**: 114–127.

Dodds C. *Anaesthesia for the Geriatric Patient.* 1993; Bailliére Tindall, London.

Hutton P, Cooper GM, James III FM and Butterworth IV JF, Eds. *Fundamental Principles and Practice of Anaesthesia.* Martin Dunitz ltd, UK 2002 IABN 1-899066-57-8. Chapter 70.

Muravchick S. Preoperative assessment of the elderly patient. *Anesthesiol Clin North America* 2000; **18**: 71–89.

Muravchick S. The elderly outpatient: current anesthetic implications. *Curr Opin Anaesthesiol* 2002; **15**: 621–625.

Chapter 3

Anaesthetic pharmacology in the elderly

> **Key points**
> - Initial distribution of drugs is often impaired.
> - Protein binding is less efficient.
> - Excretion of water-soluble drugs or metabolites is reduced.
> - Clearance of highly extracted drugs decreases with liver blood flow.
> - Inter-individual variability increases with age.
> - Titration to effect is mandatory.
> - Always favour the shortest acting and most titrable drugs.

Peri-operative anaesthetic complications in the elderly are mainly overdosing during induction of general anaesthesia, haemodynamic instability throughout the procedure and undetected aspiration of gastric content in the post-anaesthetic care unit (PACU) due to poor recovery. Only a good knowledge of the changes induced by ageing on the pharmacology of anaesthetic drugs may optimize the whole course of anaesthesia and recovery.

3.1 Changes induced by ageing on the pharmacology of anaesthetic drugs

3.1.1 Pharmacokinetics

3.1.1.1 Distribution
In the elderly, a reduction in lean body mass and total body water and an increase in fat modify drug distribution. Those changes are more important in males than in females. The volume of distribution at steady state of highly lipid-soluble drugs is markedly increased in aged individuals, which lowers their plasma concentration and delays

their elimination. On the contrary, less lipid-soluble drugs (morphine) have a smaller volume of distribution in the elderly, and see their elimination quickened in this population.

The so-called greater 'sensitivity' of aged patients to the action of many drugs can in some cases be related to a reduction in the initial volume of distribution or of the initial distribution clearance. In elderly patients compared with younger ones, the same dose will generate a markedly higher plasma concentration and thus a greater pharmacological effect.

Plasma albumin concentration tends to decrease with age, and even if the albumin plasma concentration remains normal, structural protein changes may lead to a reduced efficiency in albumin binding sites. At the same time, many chronically administered drugs that are seemingly not dangerous may compete with the anaesthetic agents on those sites and thus increase their unbound fraction. On the contrary, alpha$_1$-acid-glycoprotein (which links basic drugs such as opioids) concentration is increased in many situations, such as inflammation or cancer, frequently present in the elderly.

3.1.1.2 Elimination

3.1.1.2.1 Hepatic metabolism

Up to about 50 years of age, the liver represents a fairly constant fraction of total body weight (around 2.5%). After 50 years of age, this proportion is progressively reduced to reach only 1.6% at 90 years. Liver blood flow also decreases with age, in about 0.3 to 1.5% every year. Thus, at 65 years, the liver blood flow has lost an average 40% of its value at 25 years. The elimination clearance of highly extracted drugs (etomidate, ketamine, flumazenil, morphine, fentanyl, sufentanil, naloxone, lidocaïne, etc.) is thereby reduced in the aged population.

Hepatic drugs metabolism is achieved through two major processes: phase I (oxidation, reduction, hydrolysis) and phase II (acetylation, conjugation) reactions. Phase I reactions are mainly carried out by microsomal mono-oxygenases which include the P450 cytochromes (CYP450). Most studies agree that the liver metabolizing capacities are not modified by ageing when phase II reactions are activated. For example, the intrinsic clearance of conjugated agents is not modified, but their elimination clearance will usually be reduced because it depends on hepatic blood flow.

Changes over time in phase I reactions are more controversial. Age does not appear as an independent covariate for the mean clearance value, but increases the inter-individual variability of this parameter.

3.1.1.2.2 Renal excretion

Most anaesthetic agents are lipid soluble, thus they are filtered by the glomeruli and immediately undergo a complete tubular reabsorption which precludes their renal elimination. The kidney will excrete only their more hydro-soluble metabolites. Some metabolites (such as morphine-6-glucuronide) are pharmacologically active and their retention may prolong the pharmacological effect of the native compound due to decreased renal function. Similarly, some muscle relaxants are eliminated at least in part through the kidneys. Their clearance will be reduced in the elderly.

3.1.2 Transfer to the effect site

Modelling studies based on the observation of differences between the time course of effect of numerous drugs and the evolution of their plasma concentration have led to the establishment of an 'effect site concentration' closely related to the time course of effect and which can be calculated from the plasma concentration via a transfer rate constant. Frequently, in the elderly, the transfer of anaesthetic drugs from the plasma to the biophase is delayed. This may explain a delayed onset and a delayed recovery even when pharmacokinetics is not modified by ageing.

3.1.3 Pharmacodynamics

The central nervous system is the target of nearly all anaesthetic agents, and consequently all changes over time in this system will directly influence the handling of anaesthetic drugs in elderly population. The main effects of age on the central nervous system are

- *an overall depletion in neurotransmitters* (catecholamines, dopamine, tyrosine, serotonin) and
- *a selective attrition of cortical neurons*, with a general reduction in the density of neurons, leading to the disappearance of about 30% of the cerebral mass by the age of 80. The cerebral blood flow undergoes a similar reduction, as well as the cerebral oxygen consumption.

3.2 Influence of age on the pharmacology of specific anaesthetic drugs

3.2.1 Hypnotics

Summary table, hypnotics
• Reduce induction doses of thiopental, propofol and etomidate and titrate to effect.
• Dramatically reduce midazolam doses.
• Haemodynamic consequences are enhanced and delayed in propofol induction.
• Propofol decrement time is not prolonged.
• Minimum alveolar concentration (MAC) of all volatile agents decreases with age.

Intravenous hypnotics have little in common as far as biochemistry or pharmacokinetics are concerned. They interfere with the gamma aminoglutamic acid (GABA) receptor albeit at different binding sites. Although all intravenous hypnotics can be used for induction of anaesthesia, only propofol is commonly used for maintenance. Apart from etomidate, all have haemodynamic consequences markedly increased in the elderly.

Volatile halogenated hypnotics have very similar pharmacodynamic effects. However, these differ in their pharmacokinetics.

3.2.1.1 Thiopental

Many studies have demonstrated a reduction in thiopental requirements for induction of anaesthesia in elderly patients when compared with in young adults. Thiopental induction dose should be reduced in the elderly mostly because of pharmacokinetic changes altering the initial distribution of the drug. Thiopental should always be administered slowly in the elderly, so much so that even when all the factors known to influence the size of the induction dose are considered, a pronounced inter-individual variability still exists, which makes necessary to adjust the dose according to the observed effect in every single patient.

3.2.1.2 Propofol

Propofol has become one of the most popular hypnotic agents for induction as well as for maintenance of anaesthesia. Nevertheless, in the aged population, its use has been limited owing to its haemodynamic effects. In as early as 1986, it was observed that, in the elderly, the doses necessary to obtain a loss of consciousness were lower and the incidence of apnoeas and hypotension was increased.

Age-related changes in propofol pharmacokinetics include alterations in initial distribution (decreased initial volume and/or impaired rapid inter compartment clearance) leading to higher plasma concentration and an increased effect of the same induction dose and a reduction in elimination clearance mainly due to a decrease in hepatic blood flow buffered by extra hepatic metabolism. On the contrary, propofol elimination is not delayed in the elderly. When administering propofol as a target controlled infusion (TCI) for induction and maintenance of anaesthesia in the elderly, which improves propofol safety profile in this population, it is important to ascertain that the model implemented in the TCI device includes age as a covariate (Figure 3.1).

Pharmacodynamic studies have shown that the concentration–effect relationship was only moderately modified in the elderly whereas the transfer time to the effect site remains unchanged.

Propofol is a potent vasodilator and numerous publications have outlined the risk of hypotension when using this drug in elderly patients. Thus, for the same hypnotic effect, the haemodynamic effect will

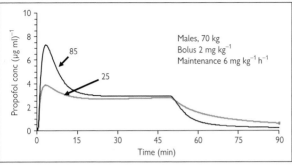

Figure 3.1 Time course of action of propofol effect site concentration when the same dosage regimen is applied to a 25-year-old or an 85-year-old individual. With the same induction dose, the peak concentration is almost doubled in the elderly, but elimination is not delayed (simulation performed with the Schnider's PK parameters set).

be increased and delayed in the elderly when compared with young subjects. It is therefore particularly important to titrate propofol to effect in order to give only the required dose and no more. TCI may help. As far as drug interactions are concerned, the adjunction of opioids to propofol for induction of anaesthesia does not allow any important reduction in the propofol dose, but potentates the drop in systolic blood pressure (SBP) and may lead to major hypotension in the absence of adrenergic stimuli.

3.2.1.3 Etomidate
Haemodynamic stability is a major advantage of etomidate, and this feature makes it very popular among anaesthetists for induction of anaesthesia in elderly patients. Despite this fact, very few studies about etomidate pharmacology in the elderly are available. The decreased etomidate dose requirements in the elderly are mainly due to changes in etomidate pharmacokinetics rather than altered brain responsiveness. The initial etomidate volume of distribution decreases significantly with increasing age (by 42% between age 22 and 80) yielding a higher initial blood concentration in the elderly following any given dose. Etomidate clearance also decreases with age, following the reduction in liver blood flow. However, the consequences of an overdose are weak, except for short procedures in which it may lead to delayed recovery.

3.2.1.4 Midazolam
Midazolam is a benzodiazepine with an intermediate clearance that is dependent both on hepatic blood flow and on the intrinsic clearance, and it has a short elimination half-life (around 2 hours).

In daily practice, it is well recognized that the dose of any benzodiazepine required for achieving a specific sedative or hypnotic end point in most elderly patients is smaller than that required in younger patients. Factors, such as midazolam central compartment volume, plasma protein binding and volume of distribution, that could influence the induction dose requirement are not affected, or only slightly affected, by the ageing process. These results suggest that the lower doses needed in the elderly are mainly attributable to pharmacodynamic changes, and profound alterations in the midazolam concentration–effect relationship have been demonstrated in the elderly. Midazolam should be used with extreme caution, if at all, for pre-medication and conscious sedation in this population as doses as low as 0.5 mg may be responsible for apnoea.

3.2.1.5 *Volatile agents*
Ageing reduces the MAC of all volatile anaesthetic agents (Figure 3.2).

Sevoflurane may be used to induce anaesthesia in the elderly, with a good haemodynamic stability probably mainly because of a progressive induction when compared with a bolus dose of intravenous drug.

Even if clinical studies are currently controversial, the preconditioning ability of volatile agents to myocardial, brain or kidney hypoxia may be of interest in this population.

Desflurane is the least lipid soluble of all volatile halogenated agents, and as such it is the most titrable and the most rapidly eliminated agent. It is therefore a drug of choice in the elderly. In the presence of opioids, no deleterious sympathetic stimulation is observed, and this drug, like sevoflurane, is associated with good haemodynamic stability.

3.2.1.6 *Nitrous oxide*
Nitrous oxide, a very common adjuvant of many general anaesthesias, should be used with caution in the elderly. This drug decreases the myocardial contractility and at the same time induces a stimulation of endogenous catecholamines. Most of the time, the haemodynamic consequences are minimal. Nevertheless, specifically in elderly patients with a cardiac condition, the use of nitrous oxide may lead to severe hypotension. This cause should be suggested when at the beginning of maintenance an unexplained hypotension is observed.

3.2.2 **Opioids**

Summary table, opioids
• Pharmacokinetic changes have very few clinical consequences.
• Increased central nervous system sensitivity conveys the need for reducing the opioid concentrations by 50%.
• Titration to effect is best achieved with remifentanil TCI.
• In the post-operative period, morphine titration to effect can be improved by patient controlled analgesia (PCA).

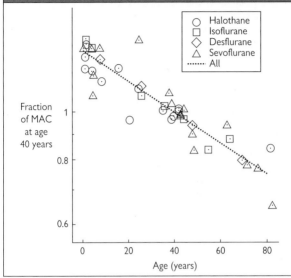

Figure 3.2 Reduction in MAC for volatile agents as a function of age

Ever since 1971, the need for reducing morphine dose with increasing age was outlined. Opioids are currently used in the vast majority of surgical patients and a poor understanding of their pharmacology may lead to serious haemodynamic or adverse respiratory events specifically in the elderly.

3.2.2.1 *Fentanyl*

Despite a worldwide use of this agent in elderly patients, fentanyl pharmacology has not been extensively studied in this population. Fentanyl is lipid soluble with a large volume of distribution at steady state and a high clearance dependent on liver blood flow. Whatever the pharmacokinetic alterations, they do not induce important changes in fentanyl plasma concentrations. Bjorkman, using a physiological model, has been able to demonstrate that after a bolus dose, the difference in a simulated plasma peak concentration was less than 3% when a 35-year-old individual was compared with a 90-year-old individual. He also stated that the reduction in clearance (liver blood flow) with age should induce a prolonged fentanyl elimination half-life in the aged.

Figure 3.2 is reproduced from Eger, E.I., *et al.* (2001). Age, minimum alveolar anesthetic concentration-awake, *Anesthesia and Analgesia*. **93**:947–53, with permission from Lippincott, Williams and Wilkins.

Nevertheless, clinical studies have clearly outlined the need to reduce fentanyl doses with increasing age. As with all other opioids, this is due to a marked increase in sensitivity to fentanyl drug effect in the elderly. These pharmacodynamic changes suggest that fentanyl doses should be decreased by 50% in aged patients.

3.2.2.2 *Alfentanil*

Alfentanil pharmacokinetics differ from that of other piperidine derivatives in that its rather low clearance is dependent both on liver blood flow and on hepatic enzyme activity. As such, it varies with the status of its metabolizing enzymes, CYP 450. Thus, alfentanil clearance is reduced by co-administered drugs (i.e. erythromycine), but may be increased by enzyme inducers, and is subject to pharmacogenetic modulation and hormonal impregnation influence. All these factors will blunt the effect of ageing on alfentanil pharmacokinetics and the results of the studies will depend highly on the population involved because the number of patients in these pharmacokinetics studies is usually low. This explains the discrepancies between the different approaches to alfentanil pharmacokinetics in the elderly. It seems that alfentanil pharmacokinetics do not depend on sex in younger patients but that ageing (menopause?) leads to a reduction in alfentanil clearance in women but not in men.

Alfentanil doses, as fentanyl doses, should be reduced by about 50% in the elderly, mostly for pharmacodynamic reasons.

3.2.2.3 *Sufentanil*

The influence of age on sufentanil pharmacokinetics has mainly been described in two studies both of which concluded that sufentanil pharmacokinetics parameters were not affected by ageing, with the exception of a reduced initial volume of distribution leading to a higher plasma peak concentration in elderly patients. Even if we lack data on the pharmacodynamics of sufentanil in the elderly, it seems reasonable to extrapolate those from fentanyl, alfentanil and morphine and conclude that the sufentanil dose should be reduced by 50% in this population.

3.2.2.4 *Remifentanil*

The influence of ageing on remifentanil behaviour has been described in details by Minto and others in a population pharmacokinetics/pharmacodynamics model including individuals who are more than 80 years old. Remifentanil pharmacokinetics in elderly individuals is characterized by a decreased initial volume of distribution, resulting in higher initial plasma concentrations following a bolus dose. Concurrently, remifentanil clearance, which is independent from hepatic function and renal blood flow but depends on the number and efficiency of tissue esterases, was decreased by about 30% from age 20 to 80.

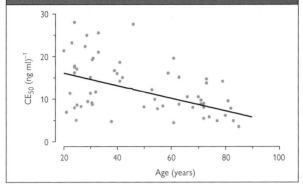

Figure 3.3 Progressive reduction with age of remifentanil CE50 for EEG effect

The transfer rate from the effect site, k_e0 was reduced with increasing age, hinting at a delayed onset of action. Moreover, the central nervous system is more sensitive to the effect of remifentanil: the concentration required to induce 50% of EEG depression (CE_{50}) was halved in 80-year-old patients when compared with that in young adults (Figure 3.3).

Whatever his or her lean body mass, an 80-year-old patient would require approximately half the dose of a 20-year-old to reach the same EEG peak effect. This end point would be delayed in the elderly (approximately 1 minute at 20 years and 2 minutes at 80 years). This adjustment in the initial bolus dose is due to pharmacodynamic changes (decreased CE_{50}). The adjustment in bolus dose for age is far more important than the adjustment in bolus dose for body weight.

The infusion rate required to maintain a constant EEG effect in an 80-year-old person is approximately one-third of that required in a 20-year-old. Again, the adjustment for age is far more important than the adjustment for body weight. This reduction in infusion rate is based on both pharmacokinetics (decreased clearance with age) and pharmacodynamics considerations (decreased CE_{50} with age).

Thus, owing to its titrability and absence of lingering effect, remifentanil appears like a very useful drug in elderly patients, provided its dosage is carefully titrated to effect. This can optimally be achieved through a target controlled remifentanil infusion. Inadequate understanding of remifentanil pharmacology in the aged patient may lead to dangerous but avoidable haemodynamic depression.

Figure 3.3 is reproduced from Minto, C.F., Schinder, T.W., Egan, T.D., *et al.* (1997). Influence of Age and Gender on the Pharmacokinetics and Pharmacodynamics of Remifentanil. *Anesthesiology.* **86**: 10–23, with permission from Lippincott, Williams and Wilkins.

3.2.2.5 *Morphine*

Morphine volume of distribution at steady state in elderly subjects is only half that of in younger patients; this difference is derived from reductions in both central and peripheral compartments. Plasma clearance is also reduced. These changes in morphine pharmacokinetics are amplified by the retention of morphine active metabolites morphine-3- and morphine-6-glucuronide, due to the physiological reduction in glomerular filtration rate in the aged. These findings suggest that the reported increased sensitivity of elderly subjects to the analgesic effects of morphine may be due at least in part to altered disposition of the drug.

Morphine pharmacodynamic data are lacking, but considering the results obtained with other opioids, it is recommended to reduce the amount of the first analgesic dose of morphine in the elderly, and to titrate further doses to effect. As often as possible, morphine PCA is appropriate in this population.

3.2.3 **Muscle relaxants**

Summary table, muscle relaxants
<ul><li>Onset is slower and duration is usually prolonged.</li><li>Atracurium and cisatracurium duration of action are not modified by ageing.</li><li>Inter-individual variability is increased, and monitoring is mandatory.</li><li>Transfer to and from the effect site is delayed.</li><li>Favour neuromuscular blocking agents (NMBAs) with non-organ elimination and ascertain that no residual paralysis is present prior to sending the patient to the PACU.</li></ul>

3.2.3.1 *Clinical findings*

The onset of action of NMBAs is usually prolonged in the elderly, irrespective of the study drug.

The duration of action of maintenance doses of rocuronium and vecuronium is significantly prolonged in the elderly, whereas that of atracurium doses is not. The maintenance infusion rate of mivacurium required to ensure adequate muscle relaxation is lower in elderly patients.

Recovery from muscle relaxation is usually delayed in elderly patients. Thus, the recovery index from 25 to 75% recovery of twitch height is increased by 60% (39–62 minutes) for pancuronium, 230% (15–49 minutes) for vecuronium, 62% (13–21 minutes) for rocuronium, 42% (5.5–7.8 minutes) for mivacurium. On the contrary, recovery from muscle relaxation is not modified by ageing for atracurium and cisatracurium.

3.2.3.2 Pharmacokinetic changes

3.2.3.2.1 Steroid compounds

Muscle relaxants with a steroid structure (pancuronium, vecuronium, rocuronium) are mainly eliminated by the liver through metabolism and biliary excretion, and partially excreted in the urine. They are poorly bound to plasma proteins. These large molecules are highly ionized regardless of pH, which limits their distribution to the extra-cellular compartment. As a consequence, their volume of distribution remains unchanged or slightly decreases with ageing.

Vecuronium is scarcely metabolized, with 40% excreted unchanged in the bile and 30% in the urine. A limited amount of the drug (30%) is deacetylated in the liver with one active metabolite. As both liver blood flow and glomerular filtration rate are reduced in the elderly, vecuronium clearance is reduced by approximately 30% in this population, without any modification in the volumes of distribution.

The elimination of rocuronium is very similar to that of vecuronium with approximately 75% eliminated in the bile and 10% in the urine. A little rocuronium undergoes deacetylation, and no significantly active metabolites are produced. Rocuronium clearance is also reduced by 30% in the elderly.

Therefore, usual pharmacokinetic parameters for steroid NMBAs are significantly but moderately modified by ageing, with a trend towards reduction in both clearance (around 30%) and distribution volumes (around 25%). These modifications have been proposed to explain prolonged duration of action, but this prolongation (at least 60%) appears important when compared with the kinetic changes.

3.2.3.2.2 Benzylisoquinoliniums

The currently available benzylisoquinoliniums include atracurium, mivacurium and cisatracurium. Atracurium and mivacurium are mixtures of stereoisomers with varying potencies and pharmacokinetics. Atracurium is a mixture of ten isomers, one of them being cisatracurium.

Like steroid NMBAs, benzylisoquinoliniums are big molecules which do not cross lipophilic barriers. Their distribution volumes are therefore in the same order of magnitude than that of the steroid compounds. Distribution volumes of benzylisoquinoliniums are slightly enhanced in elderly patients. This may be due to a potential decrease in plasma protein binding in this population, these compounds being more extensively protein bound than the steroids.

Metabolism or hydrolysis of benzylisoquinolinium compounds is quite diversified. Atracurium and cisatracurium undergo spontaneous degradation through Hofmann elimination and ester hydrolysis. This process accounts for about 83% of cisatracurium elimination clearance, but only for about 40% of atracurium total elimination clearance. The fraction of atracurium which does not undergo

Hofmann elimination is probably metabolized mainly in the liver. If atracurium total elimination clearance is not modified by ageing, its organ clearance is reduced, but this reduction is counterbalanced by an enhancement of non-organ clearance.

The main mivacurium isomers are metabolized by plasma pseudo-cholinesterases and the *cis-cis* isomer has a much lower clearance. In a letter to the *British Journal of Anaesthesia*, a decrease in pseudocholinesterase activity in elderly patients when compared with that in younger ones, though the activity remained in the normal range, was reported. This observation, which has not been confirmed by a full paper, might contribute to the reduced *trans-trans* and *cis-trans* isomers clearances.

3.2.3.3 *Effect site concentration*

Muscle blood flow has been suggested as a factor which influences delivery of drugs to the end plate. Regional blood flows, including muscle blood flow, are reduced in the elderly. Therefore a more important concentration gradient between the effect site and the plasma in elderly patients may exist, which is illustrated by a lower exit rate constant k_e0 in the aged. The slow onset and longer duration of action of most NMBAs in elderly patients, poorly explained by the scarce changes in elimination kinetics, might correspond to this phenomenon. When cisatracurium was studied, the time to maximum block was more rapid in young patients compared with elderly ones, owing to a reduction in k_e0 with age.

3.2.3.4 *Pharmacodynamics*

So far, all the clinical changes in NMBA behaviour in elderly patients have been explained by pharmacokinetic but not pharmacodynamic alterations. Plasma concentrations corresponding to a fixed degree of paralysis are not modified by ageing, and the concentration–response relationships remain usually unchanged suggesting that the ageing process has no influence on the pharmacodynamic component of NMBA behaviour.

3.2.3.5 *NMBA antagonists*

The use of NMBA antagonists such as neostigmine or edrophonium should be widely recommended in the elderly. The onset of action of neostigmine is often delayed, its effects are longer lasting possibly owing to a reduced elimination with impaired renal function and thus the dose requirements are increased. The incidence of cardiac dysrhythmias after injection of neostigmine is increased. No information is currently available on the interest of the new antagonist of the steroid NMBA Sugammadex in elderly patients but its original action sounds interesting in this population.

3.3 Conclusion

Ageing induces changes in both the pharmacokinetics and the pharmacodynamics of anaesthetic agents. These changes are not similar whatever the agent or its class, and their knowledge is necessary to adequately design any anaesthetic protocol in this population. As ageing progresses, inter-individual variability increases. Therefore, it is appropriate to choose drugs with a rapid onset and a short duration of action in the aged in order to carefully titrate their doses to the desired effect and avoid unwanted side effects, mainly haemodynamic. The way the drugs are handled in this population is much more important than the choice of the drug alone, and many dosing schemes should rather be adapted to the patient's age than to his/her weight.

Further reading

Bjorkman S, Wada DR and Stanski DR. Application of physiologic models to predict the influence of changes in body composition and blood flows on the pharmacokinetics of fentanyl and alfentanil in patients. *Anesthesiology* 1998; **88**: 657–667.

Eger EI. Age, minimum alveolar anesthetic concentration, and minimum alveolar anesthetic concentration-awake. *Anesth Analg* 2001; **93**: 947–953.

Jacobs JR, Reves JG, Marty J, White WD and Bai SA. Aging increases pharmacodynamic sensitivity to the hypnotic effects of midazolam. *Anesth Analg* 1995; **80**: 143–148.

Kazama T, Ikeda K, Morita K, Kikura M, Doi M, Ikeda T, Kurita T and Nakajima Y. Comparison of the effect site k_e0 of propofol for blood pressure and EEG bispectral index in elderly and younger patients. *Anesthesiology* 1999; **90**: 1517–1527.

Minto CF, Schnider TW and Shafer SL. Pharmacokinetics and pharmacodynamics of remifentanil. 2. Model application. *Anesthesiology* 1997; **86**: 24–33.

Minto CF, Schnider TW, Egan TD, Young E, Lemmens HJM, Gambus PL, Billard V, Hoke JF, Moore KHP, Hermann DJ, Muir KT, Mandema JW and Shafer SL. Influence of age and gender on the pharmacokinetics and pharmacodynamics of remifentanil. I. Model development. *Anesthesiology* 1997; **86**: 10–23.

Passot S, Servin F, Pascal J, Charret F, Auboyer C and Molliex S. A comparison of target- and manually controlled infusion propofol and etomidate/desflurane anesthesia in elderly patients undergoing hip fracture surgery. *Anesth Analg* 2005; **100**: 1338–1342.

Schnider TW, Minto CF, Gambus PL, Andresen C, Goodale DB, Shafer SL, Youngs EJ: The influence of method of administration and covariates on the pharmacokinetics of propofol in adult volunteers. *Anesthesiology* 1998; **88**: 1170–1182.

Schnider TW, Minto CF, Shafer SL, Gambus PL, Andresen C, Goodale DB and Youngs EJ. The influence of age on propofol pharmacodynamics. *Anesthesiology* 1999; **90**: 1502–1516.

Scott JC and Stanski DR. Decreased fentanyl/alfentanil dose requirement with increasing age: a pharmacodynamic basis. *J Pharmacol Exp Ther* 1987; **240**: 159–166.

Sorooshian SS, Stafford MA, Eastwood NB, Boyd AH, Hull CJ and Wright PM: Pharmacokinetics and pharmacodynamics of cisatracurium in young and elderly adult patients. *Anesthesiology* 1996; **84**: 1083–1091.

Chapter 4

Pre-operative assessment and preparation of elderly patients undergoing major surgery

Key points

- Age as such is not a good predictor of surgical risk.
- Physiological age-related changes increase the risks of surgery and anaesthesia.
- Co-morbidities increase with age.
- Anaesthetic plan for surgery in elderly is a challenge.
- Aim of assessment is to identify within the composite elderly patient what integrated responses are critically reduced, or have failed, and then to systematically review individual organ systems for functional reserve.
  - Incidence of ischaemic heart disease and valve disease increases with age and is associated with increased morbidity and mortality.
  - Chest disease is common in the elderly, and pulmonary complications are more common in the post-operative period.
- Hepatic insufficiency usually results in a poor surgical outcome.
- Renal insufficiency associated with uraemia increases risk.
- Presence of interval delirium or confusion indicates a very high risk of post-operative cognitive impairment and general anaesthetic or sedation should be avoided.
- Before emergency surgery, there may not be time for complete evaluation and correction of risk factors.
- Life saving treatment can proceed without consent.
- Advance directives before surgery should be documented, and the name of the patient's surrogate should be recorded.

Age as such is not a good predictor of surgical risk but certain co-morbidities that become more common with ageing and physiological age-related changes may increase the risks. Risk assessment and stratification is essential to formulate proper management strategies but it is a challenge. There are different approaches to assessing operative risk from overall medical status schemes to those which incorporate both physiology and the type of operation. Risk can also be organ specific such as cardiovascular, respiratory, neurological and so on. The prevalence of disease in elderly patients who need surgery is even higher than for elderly population in general. Emergency surgery is one of the most important factor influencing surgical outcomes in elderly. The primary aim of the assessment is to identify within the composite elderly patient what integrated responses are critically reduced, or have failed, and then to systematically review individual organ systems for functional reserve. It is important to decide what can be done to optimize the patient's condition for the planned surgery or to modify the operative plan if the patient is unlikely to survive the peri-operative period. However, before emergency surgery, there may not be time for complete evaluation and correction of risk factors. Pre-operative evaluation may include consultations with a medical or geriatric specialist, with social workers, discharge planners or psychiatrists.

The surgical and anaesthetic procedures including benefits and possible complications are explained to the patient and the patient is asked to sign an informed consent. If a patient cannot understand the surgical risks and benefits because of dementia, delirium, shock, intoxication or other reasons, permission for surgery may be granted according to the patient's advance directives or by a surrogate (a person appointed by statute to make health care decisions for another person). In cases of extreme emergency, lifesaving treatment often proceeds without consent. Advance directives (e.g. living wills, durable power of attorney for health care) are completed while a patient still has the capacity to make health care decisions. Before surgery, these directives should be documented, and the name of the patient's surrogate should be recorded.

There are different scoring systems that might help predict which patients are at risk from post-operative complications, but they generally have poor positive predictability. The decision as to whether to proceed with surgery is based on a consideration of the risks of surgery, the risks of delay to allow for further investigation or improvement and the risks of not proceeding at all. In elderly patients with severe cardiorespiratory disease, the life expectancy due to their disease may be shorter than that due to the planned surgery.

Pre-operative assessment is done using a structured approach (see Box 4.1) which includes the history, a functional reserve assessment

Box 4.1 **Structured approach of pre-assessment**

- History.
- Review of organ system by clinical examinations.
- Investigations based on assessment of functional reserve of various organs especially cardiovascular and respiratory systems.
- Investigations are required when significant symptoms and signs are new or old and evolving or severe.

and a review of organ systems. An assessment of functional reserve and review of organ systems centred on the cardiovascular and respiratory systems including clinical examination, directed by history, are performed. Where significant symptoms and signs are new, or old and evolving, or severe, further investigations may be required.

4.1 **History**

A history of general health, drug, allergies and anaesthetic are noted. The elderly often use several drugs concurrently that may cause problems peri-operatively. At least half of chronically ill patients make errors when they report their drug use and compliance; hence the health care professional concerned should be asked to confirm drug use.

4.2 **Assessment of functional reserve**

At present there are two systems that provide some insight into functional reserve: metabolic equivalence and the use of the American Society of Anesthesiology (ASA) status.

4.2.1 **Metabolic equivalence**

Major surgery generates a strong systemic inflammatory response that is associated with a rise in oxygen requirements from an average of 110 ml min^{-1} m^{-2} at rest to an average of 170 ml min^{-1} m^{-2} in the post-operative period. Inability to meet this rise in post-operative requirements creates an oxygen debt, the magnitude and duration of which correlate with the incidence of organ failure and death.

The elderly patient who has limited cardiorespiratory reserve may be unable to increase their cardiac output and oxygen delivery in order to meet this oxygen debt in the post-operative period. This functional limitation is likely to be evident in the pre-operative period and is frequently assessed as the number of Metabolic Equivalents (METS) that the patient can achieve. Metabolic equivalence is based on the calculation of the basal oxygen requirement of a 40-year-old male of 70 kg at rest (about 3.5 ml kg^{-1} min^{-1}) and then increasing his workload while recording the increases in oxygen uptake. An ability to perform exercise at greater than 4 METS is associated with a low risk of complications. An inability to climb two flights of stairs has a good positive predictive value for the development of complications. METS may be objectively measured by tests such as electrocardiogram (ECG) exercise testing or through questionnaires such as the Duke Activity status. However the difficulty remains in assessing functional capacity in those patients whose daily activities are limited by arthritis, blindness or previous cerebrovascular disease

4.2.2 **ASA status**

The ASA's physical status classification is based entirely on the identification of significant organ system dysfunction and the severity of functional impairment, and it has been shown to be a significant predictor of morbidity and mortality in surgical patients. It is used widely to classify the severity of surgical patients and to evaluate the risk related to surgical outcomes. The goal of the system is to assess the overall physical status of the patient before surgery. It is easily applied and communicated, which makes it practical to use; however, ASA lacks specificity, which leads to inconsistent ratings between anaesthetists and imprecise clinical interpretation. Indeed, the lack of precision for such a commonly used measure has resulted in numerous inquiries to the ASA. The ASA classification remains a very good predictor of outcome in the elderly. However, it does not include patient's age, type of surgery to be performed, physical and mental activities which are factors that largely affect the outcome in elderly patients.

4.3 **POSSUM**

Physiological and Operative Severity Score for the enUmeration of Mortality and morbidity (POSSUM) involves physiological as well as operative variables to calculate the risk of morbidity and mortality of surgical patients. Age is included in the physiological portion and the score increases with advancing age. The operative score includes variables such as operative magnitude, predicted blood loss, timing of operation, whether elective or emergency. POSSUM is a comprehensive tool that examines pre-operative and intra-operative variables. It is suggested that POSSUM overestimates the mortality rate in lower-risk patients but still regarded as the most appropriate scoring system available for assessing risk in non-cardiac surgical patients.

4.4 **Review of organ systems (systemic assessment)**

4.4.1 **Cardiovascular system**

The incidence of ischaemic heart disease and valve disease increases with age and is associated with an increased morbidity and mortality.

A history of exercise limitation may be absent in patients whose disease, for instance severe arthritis or blindness, prevents normal daily activities such as shopping. A high degree of suspicion is aroused in such patients and the use of investigations to provide these answers becomes necessary. The most useful investigation remains the ECG with many of the elderly displaying a significant abnormality, but it may be misinterpreted in approximately 25% of patients. Echocardiography is another highly useful modality in assessing the function of the myocardium, and in cases in which there is a concern about valvular dysfunction.

Cerebrovascular disease especially of the vertebral and carotid arteries has to be assessed not only for patients for carotid endarterectomy, but also for patients in which flexion or extension of the neck is likely. Prone positioning and extension for a rigid endoscopy are two high-risk manoeuvres if atheroma is compromising cerebral blood flow. The ability of the patient to look up from a chair without going dizzy is as good a test as any.

Autonomic function is assessed to identify the risk of reflex dysfunction, for instance postural hypotension or a poor response to acute hypovolaemia, reduced gut motility or disordered temperature homeostasis. The dearth of tests of autonomic function that can identify pre-symptomatic failure is a major limitation to pre-assessment.

Exercise testing for ischaemia remains valuable and, in cases in which there is limitation of movement, an inotrope-induced stress test is a suitable alternative. More complex investigations such as dipyridamole thallium scanning, trans-oesophageal echo or Holter monitoring may be helpful.

Many elderly patients will be taking drugs for the treatment of hypertension, ischaemic heart disease and heart failure. It is important that these drugs are given on the day of surgery and not omitted due to fact that the patient is nil-by-mouth. All drugs should be continued in the peri-operative period because withdrawal may actually be harmful, for instance in the sudden cessation of β-blocker drugs. The exception to this is with angiotensin-converting enzyme (ACE) inhibitors which should be discontinued on the day of surgery. Continuation of ACE inhibitors can lead to difficulty in maintaining blood pressure during the peri-operative period. The evidence for commencement of β- blocker drugs prior to colorectal surgery is controversial. In addition there are significant logistical difficulties in commencing these drugs in an elderly population in an outpatient setting. Anticoagulants are often used in atrial fibrillation and valvular heart disease. These will need to be stopped to ensure that clotting function is normal prior to surgery, particularly if an epidural or spinal technique is used. Anti-platelet agents such as clopidogrel should also be stopped prior to epidural insertion. Recommencement of anticoagulants such as warfarin after surgery should be on the basis of the balance risk between post-operative bleeding and further thrombosis. One should keep in mind that warfarin therapy for cardiac disease is based on a long-term risk reduction.

There are risk assessment methods such as the Goldman, Detsky and Lee cardiac index for assessing risk in patients suffering from cardiovascular diseases. Readers are advised to read major textbooks for further details.

4.4.2 **Respiratory system**

Chest disease is common in the elderly, and pulmonary complications are more common in the post-operative period compared with their incidence in younger patients. A history of smoking, active chest disease, recent chest infection or hospital admissions with pulmonary symptoms suggests the need for further investigation. Smoking and chronic obstructive pulmonary disease (COPD) are both poor predictors of outcome. The most useful investigations are those of functional reserve, while specific investigations that are single 'snapshots' of a continuum are less helpful. A '6-minute walk' is a very good indicator of the patient's ability to withstand major surgery. Clearly this is of limited value in patients who have severe arthritis or blindness, but a history (with confirmation by a relative) of social activities such as shopping or dancing will support estimation of metabolic equivalence. Of the more routine investigations, arterial blood gases and chest X-ray provide useful information. Formal pulmonary function testing for peak flow rate, forced vital capacity in 1 second (FEV1) and forced vital capacity (FVC) allow an estimation of physiological reserve to be made by comparison with expected age adjusted values. The presence of reversibility following bronchodilators suggests that there is potential for improvement. A history should be sought for the presence of snoring, and observed pauses in breathing. This may be more difficult in widowed patients, but families will often have complained about the problem. Where there is a positive history, overnight oximetry is a useful investigation test to identify episodic airway collapse and to identify the median saturation when supine. The patient may be prone to post-operative sleep apnoea, particularly if opioid-based analgesia is instituted. The patient may benefit from continuous pulse-oximetry to detect night-time desaturation. Pre-operative physiotherapy and incentive spirometry may also be useful in reducing post-operative pulmonary complications. In extreme cases there may be a requirement for post-operative ventilatory support. In these cases, there may be a need to alter the surgical plan to perform less invasive surgery to reduce the metabolic demand and to maintain effective pulmonary function.

4.4.3 **Nervous system**

A history should be sought of any recent operations with particular attention being paid to the incidence of interval delirium or confusion.

This indicates a very high risk of post-operative cognitive impairment and may indicate the avoidance of a general anaesthetic or even sedation. Where there is any doubt about the state of the patient's cognition, the most practical test (see Table 4.1 and Box 4.2) applicable by anaesthetists is the mini-mental state evaluation (MMSE). The use of simpler tests is acceptable when time is pressing, but these tests cannot support a clinical diagnosis in isolation. Vision and hearing should be assessed, as should the patient's literacy before detailed explanations of procedure or technique are discussed. The competency to give informed consent also has to be investigated.

Table 4.1 Mini-mental state evaluation (MMSE) sample

Score	Section	Task
	Orientation	
5	e.g.	What is the date?
	Registration	
3	e.g.	Listen carefully. I am going to say three words. You say them back after I stop. Ready? Here they are... APPLE (pause), PENNY (pause), TABLE (pause). Now repeat those words back to me. [Repeat up to 5 times, but only score the first trial.]
	Language	
2	e.g.	What is this? [Point to a pencil or pen.]
3	e.g.	Please read this and do what it says. [Show examinee the words on the stimulus form.] CLOSE YOUR EYES.
30	Total score	

This table is only a sample of the complete MMSE, which takes about 10–15 minutes, and requires some written material for the last test.. The full MMSE can be purchased from Psychological Assessment Resources (PAR) Inc. by calling: (+1) (813) 968-3003.

Box 4.2 Score results

30–29	Normal.
28–26	Borderline cognitive dysfunction.
25–18	Marked cognitive dysfunction – may be diagnosed as demented.
<17	Severe dysfunction – severe dementia.

47

Advanced age and a history of delirium or confusion following previous surgery convey a higher risk of early post-operative cognitive dysfunction (POCD), although the incidence of POCD 1–2 years later is low. This may indicate the avoidance of a general anaesthetic if feasible. Adequacy of vision and hearing should be assessed so that the anaesthetic technique may be explained appropriately.

4.4.4 Hepatic system

Hepatic insufficiency usually results in a poor surgical outcome. Hepatic insufficiency is suspected on the basis of history and sometimes on routine pre-operative liver function tests. The only pre-operative precautions that can be taken are correction of coagulation abnormalities with vitamin K or blood products (e.g. fresh frozen plasma, coagulation concentrates).

4.4.5 Renal system

Renal insufficiency, particularly with uraemia, increases surgical risk. In the elderly, the serum creatinine level must be adjusted for age and decreased lean body mass. Pre-renal azotaemia can often be corrected with IV fluids. Peritoneal dialysis or haemodialysis may alleviate uraemia and reduce surgical risk. For all patients with renal insufficiency with normal serum creatinine but reduced creatinine clearance, dosages of renally excreted drugs must be adjusted.

4.4.6 Thrombo-embolic disease

The incidence of deep vein thrombosis is relatively higher in elderly patients undergoing general surgery and is much higher for the elderly patients undergoing hip or knee surgery, neurosurgery, open prostatectomy, or a gynaecologic cancer surgical procedure. The elderly are also at increased risk of a fatal pulmonary embolism post-operatively. Prophylactic treatment should be considered before any major surgical procedure. Patients taking warfarin or anti-platelet drugs are at increased risk of bleeding during and after surgery. However, stopping the drug may increase risk of thrombotic complications.

4.4.7 Other systems

Poorly controlled diabetes increases risk of peri-operative infection. Peri-operative stress increases production of counter-regulatory hormones that increase plasma glucose (e.g. catecholamines, cortisol, glucagon). Glucose should be monitored closely. Oral anti-hyperglycaemic drugs should be stopped at least a day before surgery (3 days for chlorpropamide). Insulin-dependent patients can be treated with an IV insulin infusion. Long-standing diabetes increases the risk of cardiovascular complications, possibly including silent myocardial ischemia. Patients should be monitored closely, and ECG should be done post-operatively.

The skin is rarely inspected pre-operatively, yet it is a mirror to so many underlying problems. Fragile, thin and bruised skin over the hands gives an indication of a poorly maintained collagen matrix and the risk of ligament damage or subluxation of joints. The bruising of vessel fragility is a sign of possible intra-operative bleeding problems or extravasation of infusions especially if they are transfused under pressure or in high volume. This pattern also warns of the risk of pressure sore formation if there are shearing forces applied on transferring the patient off and on to trolleys or tables.

Thin, frail patients have limited subcutaneous fat and poor muscle bulk. They will not be able to preserve their core temperature either on the ward or in the theatre and will not have the metabolic capacity for the necessary shivering response to restore normothermia afterwards.

Gut function is less efficient in elderly patients than in younger patients and the frequency of acid regurgitation increases in these patients. Gut motility is reduced leading to prolonged gastric emptying times and delayed entry into the small gut. The colon is similarly affected and constipation is common. These are important issues for the patient especially if the surgery is likely to be painful and opiates necessary.

4.5 **Nutritional status**

The mortality rate is significantly higher in patients who have lost more than 20% of body weight before surgery. Nutritional status is assessed by standard instruments, such as the Mini Nutritional Assessment or Subjective Global Assessment. Serum albumin is measured in patients with chronic disorders, who show signs of under-nutrition, or who have poor wound healing. A value of <3.5 g dL^{-1} indicates higher risk of complications and mortality but may not, by itself, correlate with nutritional status. Pre-operative nutritional support might offer some benefit in reducing complication rates.

4.6 **Pre-operative blood tests**

It is well known that laboratory values are not significant predictors of peri-operative complications. However, estimation of haemoglobin and platelet concentration should be carried out if they are to undergo major surgery. Tests of clotting function are unlikely to be abnormal without significant liver disease or anticoagulant therapy. Haemoglobin levels are often low. This may be due to gastrointestinal losses from the tumour site, and patients may not have sufficient haematinic stores to restore their haemoglobin levels themselves in the post-operative period. A decrease in serum albumin to <2.1 g dL^{-1}

is associated with an exponential increase in mortality. Serum urea and electrolyte values should also be obtained. Abnormal values are relatively common. Diuretic use may lead to low serum potassium values. However normal urea and creatinine values do not necessarily mean that renal function is normal. Reduced dietary intake and muscle mass mean that the respective values of urea and creatinine are lower in the elderly. In addition, renal function needs to deteriorate markedly before urea and creatinine levels are elevated beyond normal values.

The process of ageing affects all of the elderly population and becomes progressively more apparent with increasing chronological age. Increased prevalence of disease in ageing population includes cardiovascular disorders (hypertension and ischaemic coronary artery disease) and respiratory disorders. Assessment of organ system functional reserve and identification of other organs at risk is primary goal of pre-operative assessment and is essential to the formulation of a good anaesthetic plan.

Further reading

Dodds C and Allison J. Postoperative cognitive deficit in the elderly surgical patient. *Br J Anaesth* 1998; **81**: 449–462.

Guidelines for Peri-operative Cardiovascular Evaluation for Non-Cardiac Surgery. Report of the American College of Cardiology/American Heart Association Task Force on Practice Guidelines (Committee on Peri-operative Cardiovascular Evaluation for Non-Cardiac Surgery). *Circulation* 1996; **93**: 1278–1317.

Jin F and Chung F. Minimising perioperative adverse events in the elderly. *Br J Anaesth* 2001; **87**: 608–624.

Jones AG and Hunter JM. Anaesthesia in the elderly. Special considerations. *Drugs Aging* 1996; **9**: 319–331.

Priebe HJ. The aged cardiovascular risk patient. *Br J Anaesth* 2000; **85**: 763–778.

Chapter 5

Day case anaesthesia in the elderly

> **Key points**
>
> - Ambulatory anaesthesia can be a very good choice in elderly patients provided an adult can escort them home and take care of them.
> - The pre-operative anaesthesia assessment should be performed sufficiently ahead of the surgery to allow preparation and adaptation of chronic treatments.
> - Spinal anaesthesia is often associated with delayed discharge when compared with general anaesthesia using short acting agents.
> - When applicable, local anaesthesia or peripheral nerve block provide long-lasting post-operative analgesia.

5.1 Indications and limitations of day case anaesthesia in the elderly

Ambulatory anaesthesia and surgery, when surgery is compatible with it, can be an excellent choice in very old patients specifically if they are confused or disorientated since it takes them far from their usual environment for only a short while. After minor surgery, cognitive dysfunction at 7 days is more severe when elderly patients are treated as inpatients rather than as outpatients.

Nevertheless, ambulatory surgery can be considered in elderly patients only if a responsible and reasonably fit adult can escort them home and care for them until they can resume their normal activities. The husband/wife does not always fulfil these requirements. Stable ASA (American Society of Anesthesiology) physical status III patients will most of the time be accepted for ambulatory procedures but the medical team must be conscious that the incidence of complications is higher in this population.

5.2 Pre-operative assessment and preparation

In elderly outpatients, concomitant diseases (hypertension, ischaemic heart disease, history of strokes, impaired cognitive function, diabetes mellitus, etc.) and chronic treatments are the rule rather than the exception. History and physical examination will provide the best estimation of the patient's pre-operative condition. Screening laboratory tests are no more contributive in the elderly than in the rest of the population. On the contrary, laboratory tests orientated by history and physical examination will provide important information on the current status of the patient and allow if appropriate an adequate preparation for the planned surgical procedure (Box 5.1).

Nevertheless, considering the high frequency of anaemia and renal failure, haemoglobin and creatinine concentrations should be measured even in seemingly healthy patients. If the interest of chest radiographs is often questionable, specifically for minor procedures, an electrocardiogram should be obtained as a baseline assessment considering the high frequency of EKG abnormalities in this population. To be really efficient, the pre-operative assessment by the anaesthesiologist should be performed early enough before the surgery to allow this preparation and the adaptation of chronic treatments. This assessment, which will be associated with explanation of the actual course of anaesthesia and surgery and answering many fearsome questions, will reassure the patient and suppress the need for drug pre-medication. Indeed, such pre-medication may have unreliable effect and duration of action and lead to unexpected hospital admission.

5.3 Which anaesthetic protocol?

5.3.1 Conscious sedation

Associated if appropriate to a local anaesthesia provided by the surgeon, this technique, when applicable, conveys the best chance of rapid recovery and is therefore well suited to the ambulatory setting. Nevertheless it should be used with great caution taking into account the specificities of pharmacology in the elderly. An adequate monitoring, similar to the one applied during general anaesthesia, should be used.

Midazolam is difficult to handle in this population and may trigger confusion and difficulties in controlling the patient. The drug of choice is currently propofol, best administered by effect site target controlled infusion (TCI) through a device implemented with a model including age as a covariate, or by patient controlled sedation. Sedation is usually obtained with targets around 1–2 μg ml^{-1}, but titration to effect should always prevail. A growing interest is emerging now for remifentanil effect site TCI which alleviates pain without altering consciousness. Some precautions are mandatory: close intra-operative monitoring of respiratory rate and pulse oximetry (ideally non-invasive monitoring of $P_{ET}CO_2$), prophylaxis of post-operative nausea and vomitting (PONV), and when applicable, administration of analgesics to prevent post-operative pain as soon as induction of sedation or even as a pre-medication.

5.3.2 **Regional anaesthesia**

Peripheral blocks when applicable (hand surgery, cataract, etc.) are a very good choice for the elderly outpatient. They provide excellent post-operative analgesia and rapid street fitness. Even if some consensus is arising as to their use in patients taking aspirin, peripheral blocks should be used with extreme caution if at all in patients undergoing anti-platelet therapy. They remain contraindicated in patients on heparin or anticoagulants. Peripheral blocks of the lower limb are less suited to the ambulatory setting since they may impair the patient's mobility for as long as 24 hours. Central blocks and specifically spinal anaesthesia are more controversial in the elderly. Spinal anaesthesia does not provide post-operative analgesia, so it presents no advantage over general anaesthesia in this respect, and it is frequently associated specifically in male patients with difficult post-operative voiding which may prolong recovery or even lead to unanticipated hospital admission.

5.3.3 **General anaesthesia**

In these short outpatient procedures, general anaesthesia using the newest hypnotic and analgesic drugs provides excellent intra-operative titrability and rapid clear- headed recovery. The drugs of choice are propofol (consider TCI), desflurane or sevoflurane, alfentanil or remifentanil (consider TCI). A laryngeal mask is often applicable for airway control. If surgery does not require muscle relaxation, a good method to assess the adequacy of anaesthesia is to use pressure support to ensure adequate ventilation while allowing monitoring of respiratory rate.

5.4 **Post-operative care**

Despite contradictory publications, elderly patients, specifically if ASA physical status III, usually cannot bypass the post-anaesthetic care unit (PACU) after ambulatory surgery. Recovery is unspecific, but post-operative analgesia should try to avoid opioids which convey a risk of drowsiness precluding rapid discharge.

The patient and/or his/her escort should receive written as well as oral instructions about the post-operative period.

Further reading

Chung F, Mezei G and Tong D. Adverse events in ambulatory surgery. A comparison between elderly and younger patients. *Can J Anaesth* 1999; **46**: 309–321.

Flaishon R, Ekstein P, Matzkin H and Weinbroum AA. An evaluation of general and spinal anesthesia techniques for prostate brachytherapy in a day surgery setting. *Anesth Analg* 2005; **101**: 1656–1658.

Muravchick S. Preoperative assessment of the elderly patient. *Anesthesiol Clin North America* 2000 Mar; **18**(1): 71–89.

Muravchick S. The elderly outpatient: Current anesthetic implications. *Curr Opin Anaesthesiol* 2002; **15**: 621–625.

Chapter 6

Emergency anaesthesia in the elderly

Key points

- Emergency surgery in the elderly is often associated with a poor outcome.
- Conditioning the patient is important, but should not delay surgery.
- Hypovolaemia, frequent in emergency procedures in aged patients, is not well tolerated, but neither is rapid fluid loading.
- A minimal trauma may result in fractured neck of the femur which, in this situation, reflects a poor physiological status.
- New surgical techniques (colonic stent, vascular stent, etc.) are currently under investigation.

Emergency surgery is comparatively more frequent in the elderly than in younger patients, and has to be performed even in cases where elective surgery might appear unreasonable. It concerns mainly trauma surgery (fractured femoral neck, broken wrist, etc.), emergency intra-abdominal surgery (occlusive syndromes due to inguinal hernias or digestive mainly colic cancer; peritonitis), and vascular surgery (acute arterial thrombosis, ruptured aortic aneurism). It may be delayed by late discovery and the patient's general condition is often poor, worsened by hypovolaemia and interruption of chronic treatments. Pain, infection, hypotension and metabolic disorders may lead to a confused state even if dementia did not pre-exist. In the absence of family or previous medical record, the patient's medical history may be difficult to precise. For all these reasons, the outcome of emergency surgery is poorer than that of elective operations in similar patients. Nevertheless, there are no major differences between old patients undergoing emergency surgery and younger ones. They may suffer from the same traumas, and the overall care is not fundamentally different from what it can be at other ages.

6.1 Pre-operative care: conditioning of the elderly patient before emergency surgery

When an elderly patient is proposed for an emergency surgery, an overall assessment of his/her medical condition has to be done in a short period of time, depending on the nature of the case.

The pre-anaesthetic assessment of a geriatric patient who has fallen should focus as much on the causes of the fall as on its consequences. Inadvertent chronic medication overdose, vertebrobasilar arterial insufficiency leading to 'drop attack', aortic stenosis and rhythm abnormalities should be looked for.

The need to stabilize concurrent medical condition should not unduly delay the surgical act. A recent study on nearly 130,000 admissions for fractured neck of femur in Great Britain has demonstrated that delay in operation was associated with an increased risk of death, even after adjustment for co-morbidity (Bottle, BMJ 2006) (Figure 6.1).

When an elderly patient is admitted in emergency in a confused state which does not allow a proper recording of his/her medical history and chronic treatments, a careful clinical examination, EKG, blood cell count and blood chemistry should try to recognize significant factors such as coronary artery disease, aortic stenosis or anti-coagulant therapy which may modify the peri-operative management. Anti-platelet treatment, very frequent in this population, is more difficult to recognize through a rapid screening.

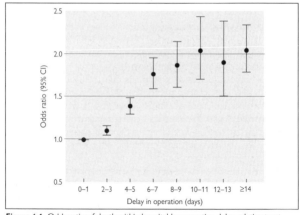

Figure 6.1 Odds ratio of death within hospital by operative delay relative to at most a day's delay, after adjustment for age, sex, deprivation, type of procedure (fixation and replacement only), and selected co-morbidities (Bottle, 2006).

Figure 6.1 is reproduced from Bottle, A., Aylin, P. (2006). Mortality associated with delay in operation after hip fracture. *British Medical Journal*, with permission from BMJ Publishing Group Ltd.

6.2 **Coping with hypovolaemia**

Hypovolaemia is very common in elderly patients presented for emergency surgery, even in the absence of bleeding or shock. The tolerance to hypovolaemia is particularly poor in elderly patients who have decreased β-receptor responsiveness, which means that to maintain an adequate cardiac output the aged heart cannot increase its heart rate, but must rely on increased ventricular filling (Franck–Starling law) and stroke volume. As a consequence, the decrease in sympathetic activity induced by both general anaesthesia and central blockade may trigger profound hypotension in this population. On the other hand, in an aged patient, rapid correction of hypovolaemia in the absence of proper monitoring, may easily lead to overloading, pulmonary oedema and heart failure. These complications will often be unmasked during the recovery period, when the vasodilatation induced by either general anaesthesia or central blockade wears off. Oesophageal Doppler ultrasonography or continuous estimations of cardiac output through an arterial line may help. In this population, early vasopressor use should be advocated.

There is no clear consensus about transfusion thresholds in the elderly. Nevertheless, considering that the majority of those patients suffer from ischaemic heart disease, and that redistribution of fluids in the post-operative period associated with some blood loss through drains will further lower the haemoglobin concentration, it seems reasonable not to allow Hb value to drop much under 100 g L^{-1} in emergency elderly patients.

6.3 **The trauma patient**

Traumas in the elderly are most often caused by falls; they can be victims of assault or attempted suicide. Because of osteoporosis, loss of muscle mass and decreased elasticity of connective tissues, the same traumatic force will generate more severe injuries in the elderly than in younger adults.

Fractured neck of the femur is the most common traumatic injury in the elderly. The causative accident is only anecdotic, and hip fracture in the elderly usually corresponds to a profound alteration of their physiological status. Its long-term mortality is high and has not been reduced in the past decades despite all the efforts and improvements in surgical techniques and anaesthesia care. Numerous studies have attempted to define the best anaesthesia technique in this situation, but no difference in outcome when comparing general and spinal anaesthesia has ever been demonstrated.

6.4 **Emergency laparotomy in the elderly**

Intra-abdominal surgical procedures that are most commonly performed in emergency on elderly patients are complications of colonic cancer (obstruction, perforation), appendicitis, cholecystitis, strangulated groin hernia and intestinal infarction. In all cases, mortality is significant (from 15 to 40%, and much more in case of acute mesenteric ischaemia), due to metabolic disorders and sepsis. Conditioning the patient before surgery must not delay the act. For example, postponing surgery beyond 24 hours after the onset of symptoms in patients with unresponsive symptoms for complete small bowel obstruction raises dramatically the risk of resection, septic shock and ultimately death. Elderly patients arrive frequently at the hospital late after the onset of symptoms.

Malignant obstruction is the most frequent cause of emergency large bowel surgery. In about 25% of the cases, the patient will undergo either Hartmann's procedure or formation of a palliative stoma. In elderly frail individuals, this stoma will never be reversed. Colonic stenting has recently been proposed with promising results as an alternative to surgery for malignant large bowel obstruction or as a temporary relief allowing delayed surgery in better conditions thus avoiding stoma.

Further reading

Bickel NA, Federman AD and Aufses AH Jr. Influence of time on risk of bowel resection in complete small bowel obstruction. *J Am Coll Surg* 2005; **201**: 847–854.

Bottle A and Aylin P. Mortality associated with delay in operation after hip fracture: Observational study. *BMJ* 2006 Apr 22; **332**(7547): 947–951.

Konttinen N and Rosenberg PH. Outcome after anaesthesia and emergency surgery in patients over 100 old. *Acta Anaesthesiol Scand* 2006; **50**: 283–289.

Venn R, Steele A and Richardson P. Randomized controlled trial to investigate influence of the fluid challenge on duration of hospital stay and perioperative morbidity in patients with hip fractures. *Br J Anaesth* 2002; **88**: 65–71.

Chapter 7

Anaesthesia for orthopaedic surgery in the elderly

Key points

- Elderly patients may have significant organ dysfunction.
  - Cardiorespiratory, renal, neurological dysfunctions and arthritis are common.
- Major joint surgery is increasingly performed.
- Pre-operative assessment is essential to optimize the disease state.
- Elderly patients may be malnourished.
- There is no single clear technique of anaesthesia.
- The use of cement during surgery is known to be associated with intra-operative morbidities.
- Tourniquet use is common during distal bone or joint surgery.
- Sedation is commonly used when regional technique is in use.
- Deep vein thrombosis (DVT) prophylaxis is necessary in patients undergoing major joint surgery.
- Antibiotics are routinely used but must be administered before tourniquet is used.
- Blood loss may be excessive especially during revision surgery and measures should be taken to minimize blood loss.
- Regional technique with opioid provides good analgesia.
- Patient controlled analgesia (PCA) with opioid is a good method but patient may not use it properly because of arthritis or impaired cognitive function.
- Prolonged use of urinary catheter should be avoided.
- Delirium is common in elderly and occurs to some degree in the vast majority of patients and anaesthesia may compound this problem.
- Early mobilization is helpful.

Elective and emergency orthopaedic surgery involves joint replacement, fixation of broken bones and the endoscopic examination of joints, but there is a huge variety of operations, ranging from minor surgery such as toe nail excision to massive revision limb and joint salvage, involving elderly patients. Significant proportions of these patients will have some degree of organ dysfunction. They are likely to suffer from rheumatoid arthritis, ankylosing spondylitis and other systemic diseases and usually receive multiple drugs. Anaesthesia for orthopaedic surgery poses particular challenges relating to the elderly patients and procedure type to the anaesthetist. An effective pre-operative assessment is of paramount importance. This chapter covers the general principles of anaesthesia relevant to orthopaedic surgery. Pre-operative preparation for surgery and anaesthesia; peri-operative management including monitoring and analgesia and post-operative management including fluid balance, critical care and recovery will be covered.

7.1 **Pre-operative preparation and assessment**

The objective of pre-operative assessment is to identify and optimize any disease state. It is important to differentiate between chronic stable disease and deteriorating clinical states which need further specialist input. Concurrent medical therapy can be checked and optimized for the surgical period with appropriate tests arranged at this stage (see Chapter 4). The majority of these patients are likely to be older and have more serious medical problems. However, the elective nature of the surgery allows time for a thorough work-up, and effective treatment can be initiated if necessary. A history of hypertension, myocardial infarction, heart failure, cerebrovascular disease and respiratory disease, renal and hepatic insufficiency should be sought. Active infection is an absolute contraindication to joint replacement and any potential source, such as urinary or dental infection, must be eliminated. Aspirin and non-steroidal anti-inflam-matory drugs are frequently the mainstays of analgesic treatment for arthritic patients, and gastritis, anaemia and platelet dysfunction may occur. Accompanying medical and orthopaedic problems, together with side effects from drug treatment, make the rheumatoid patient considerably more difficult to treat. Anti-hypertensive, other cardiac and respiratory drugs should be administered as normal on the day of surgery.

7.2 Nutritional assessment

Many elderly patients are malnourished and associated proteinaemia can adversely affect wound healing and increase the potential of post-operative complications. Aggressive post-operative nutritional protein supplementation in patients hospitalized with hip fractures has been associated with weight gain, shorter durations of hospitalization and reductions in post-operative complications. Most patients can tolerate enteral nutrition within 12–24 hours post-operatively. Oral protein supplements should be used in the vast majority of these patients because their intake in the immediate post-operative period may be diminished from baseline. If oral intake is inadequate, naso-gastric tube feeding may be effective in improving nitrogen balance and caloric intake.

7.3 Elective surgery

Elective joint replacement is now an established treatment for end-stage disease of a joint for a variety of reasons including osteoarthritis, rheumatoid arthritis, osteoporosis, metastatic lesions and avascular necrosis. Since the innovative work of Charnley in the 1960s on the development of total hip replacement, there have been many advances in design and metallurgy. As a result of increased understanding of the biomechanical principles involved in the development of prostheses, and the use of acrylic cement to transmit forces between metal and bone, joint replacement has become increasingly successful. Custom-made prostheses are also being increasingly used and are inserted without the use of cement.

7.3.1 Hip replacement surgery

Total hip arthroplasty presents a challenge (see Box 7.1) because of the age group of the typical patient and their associated co-morbidity, the complexity of the nerve supply to the hip and surrounding structures and the severity of the surgery. Most hip prostheses used are of the cemented variety. The surgery is performed in either supine or a modified lateral position using sandbags. Surgery involves insertion of an acetabulam cup and removal of the femoral head which is replaced with a femoral component. Cement called 'polymethylmethacrylate' is used to fix cup and femoral components.

There is no single clearly superior technique for either anaesthesia or post-operative analgesia but on balance of risk and benefit, the evidence points to regional anaesthesia having proven benefits over

Box 7.1 Considerations during hip surgery

- Hip surgery in the elderly is major challenge and is performed in supine or modified lateral position.
  - Hip fracture should be fixed as soon as possible to reduce pain and minimize complications as delay can lead to decline in functional status and increased medical problems.
- There is no single clear superior technique of anaesthesia.
  - Regional anaesthesia appears to have marginal benefit.
- Use of cement is common and may be associated with morbidity.
  - Cement insertion into the femoral shaft may be accompanied by sudden reduction in end tidal carbon dioxide and decrease in blood pressure.
  - Slowing of heart rate may occur.
  - Exact cause is not known but air and fat embolism are considered be major contributing factors.
- Prevention of DVT and infection are important.

general anaesthesia and systemic opioids and also to the benefits of extending regional anaesthesia–based analgesia into the post-operative recovery period. There are advantages and disadvantages of each technique.

Sedation is generally used with regional anaesthesia which is either epidural or more preferably spinal anaesthesia. The advantages of regional anaesthesia include decreased blood loss, reduced risk of deep venous thrombosis, immediate post-operative analgesia as well as prolonged post-operative analgesia, early mobilization, decreased risk of respiratory infection, less vomiting and less mental confusion in the elderly. Unfortunately there are still many surgeons and patients who do not like regional anaesthesia. These are known complications of regional techniques such as hypotension, headache, inadequate block and the like, but there are few absolute contraindications to regional techniques even though regional blocks may be sometimes difficult to perform in the elderly.

General anaesthesia may be preferred by the patient as well as the surgeon because of better cardiovascular stability and control of the airway. However, the disadvantages of general anaesthesia include risks such as slower recovery, slower mobilization, incidence of nausea and vomiting, increased incidence of post-operative cognitive dysfunction and increased risk of respiratory infection.

Revision of hip replacement surgery may take several hours; therefore, general anaesthesia is employed. A single-shot regional anaesthesia is not appropriate but a catheter-based technique is suitable in some patients although they may become uncomfortable despite the use of sedation.

Application of cement particularly after its insertion into the femoral shaft may be accompanied by a sudden reduction in end tidal carbon dioxide and decrease in blood pressure. Slowing of heart rate may occur and cardiac arrest is known to occur. It is usually attributed to toxic monomers released as the cement polymerises. The incidence was much more frequent when the technique was relatively new. Air embolism (air trapped under the cement forced into the circulation as the prosthesis is pushed into the femoral shaft) was thought to be another reason. The technique of filling cement into the shaft from the bottom upwards has reduced the incidence of adverse events but insertion can still cause embolism of fat, blood clots or marrow. Intramedullary pressure may increase above the venous pressure thus leading to embolisation of air.

Full cardiovascular monitoring is essential and a patent intravenous line with free flowing fluid should always be running.

The current evidence of best practice for hip replacement recommends either a single-shot local anaesthetic spinal with a small (100–200 mcg) dose of morphine or a general anaesthetic with minimal opioid use combined with a lumbar plexus block. Both techniques offer a good risk–benefit profile.

7.3.2 Knee replacement surgery

General anaesthesia with opioid analgesia with or without intubation (laryngeal mask airway (LMA)) is an appropriate technique. This surgery is carried out with the patient supine and a tourniquet is used. Antibiotics are administered prior to inflation of the tourniquet. Epidural or spinal anaesthesia with small dose of opiate provides good anaesthesia and post-operative analgesia. Sedation with small dose of midazolam is usually helpful to relieve anxiety caused by the noise of sawing and other instrumentation. Thorough attention to haemostasis by the surgeon is required following tourniquet release but prior to wound closure. When the tourniquet is released, acidic by-products of metabolism are released. These cause hypotension secondary to vasodilatation and negative effects on cardiac contractility. If the tourniquet is not released until the end of the surgery, the patient, on awakening, can experience pain from this cause alone.

Knee replacement surgery is very painful for the first 12 hours after surgery and a regional technique has an advantage. The pain can be lessened by combined sciatic and 'three in one' femoral sheath block. Local infiltration of local anaesthetic agent after general anaesthesia is helpful in reducing post-operative pain.

Peripheral blocks (femoral +/− sciatic block) in combination with a general anaesthetic are a practical and effective alternative to spinal or epidural block and, with fewer side effects and equal analgesic benefit, are probably the method of choice. Post-operative infusion of local anaesthetic via sciatic and femoral catheters for up to 72 hours may provide excellent analgesia (lowest pain scores and minimum rescue analgesia required); whether this improves outcome remains to be seen. Continuous or patient controlled infusions of even dilute local anaesthetics and adjuvant drugs can delay return of full motor and proprioceptive function and thus inhibit active rehabilitation at 24 hours.

The use of a tourniquet is common during some orthopaedic procedures to produce a bloodless field. Effective venous exsanguination is produced by elevating the limb or winding a rubber bandage (Esmarch bandage) followed by inflation of a tourniquet cuff to a pressure sufficient to occlude arterial supply. The tourniquet is inflated and maintained 100 mmHg higher than the systolic blood pressure. Because elderly skin is very friable and muscles and nerves can be damaged, it is important to apply fabric or cotton under the cuff. Prolonged application of tourniquet can lead to electromyographical and histological changes but they are usually reversed after deflation. The products of anaerobic metabolism in the limb are released and a bolus of acidic and hypercapnic blood is returned to the circulation. This can result in transient cardiovascular and neurological changes. The use of a tourniquet should be avoided in patients with poor peripheral circulation, crush injury, infection, sickle cell disease and so on.

7.3.3 **Shoulder surgery**

Major surgical procedures on the shoulder include replacement of joints, open surgery or repair of joint by arthroscopic approach. Surgery often involves vigorous manipulation of the joint in the semi-sitting position; hence the patient's head needs to be supported and protected. Anaesthetic techniques vary for shoulder surgery. General anaesthesia techniques vary from intubation with a reinforced tracheal tube and controlled ventilation of the patient to spontaneous ventilation via an armoured laryngeal mask airway in selected patients. Post-operative pain can be relieved by intravenous morphine through a PCA machine. Intermittent or continuous injection of local anaesthetic through a sub-arcromial catheter inserted at the end of surgery is an option for pain relief.

Regional techniques are also employed and to ensure the shoulder is completely blocked, a supraclavicular approach is necessary. The most common is the interscalene approach to the brachial plexus, which provides excellent intra-operative analgesia, decreased blood loss and good muscle relaxation for any shoulder operation. As with all regional techniques this should be performed awake and complications must be sought for and treated; the commonest include phrenic nerve palsy, Horner's syndrome, block of the recurrent laryngeal nerve and transient neuroparexia may occur. A good regional analgesia technique extending into the post-operative period improves the chances of early post-operative mobilization and physiotherapy for the shoulder joint.

Blood pressure monitors can be used on the non-operative limb or the leg. If venous access is used on the same limb as the blood pressure cuff, using a non-return valve will prevent venous blood filling up the venous cannula when the blood pressure is being recorded. A fully functional intravenous infusion line with remote injection facility should be available.

The patient is positioned in a semi-sitting position with a sandbag between the shoulders to improve surgical access. The head must be secured, as traction can pull it off the head ring and dislodgement of the tracheal tube can occur. The eyes should be well padded. All monitoring equipment must be fully functional and electro-cardiogram (ECG) and connectors are secured.

7.3.4 **Hand and distal arm surgery**

Regional anaesthesia is especially suitable for surgery on the hand and arm provided the duration of surgery is not unduly prolonged. Brachial plexus block, a peripheral nerve block or intravenous regional anaesthesia are the usual techniques used. Measures need to be taken to reduce tourniquet discomfort. If general anaesthesia is required, a simple anaesthetic technique with an laryngeal mask airway (LMA) is what is required.

7.3.5 **Foot and lower extremity surgery**

Operation on the lower leg can be accomplished with peripheral nerve block either at the level of femoral and sciatic nerves or by individual nerve blocks at the level of the knee. However, these blocks are difficult to achieve without the help of an ultrasound machine and experience and training is essential.

7.3.6 **Arthroscopic surgery**

Arthroscopic surgery is usually performed in younger patients but they are also performed in elderly patients for diagnostic purposes. All forms of anaesthesia previously described for shoulder surgery are suitable.

7.4 **Emergency surgery**

7.4.1 **Surgery for hip fracture**

Patients who undergo surgery for hip fracture are usually frail and female. Surgical aims are to fix the fracture as soon as possible, to reduce pain and minimize complications associated with prolonged bed rest. Excessive delay in surgery and delay in weight bearing may lead to decline in functional status and increased medical problems. Early repair of fracture (within 24–48 hours) is associated with a reduction in 1-year mortality and lower incidences of pressure sores, confusion and fatal pulmonary embolism (PE). However, this may not be possible in some patients who have unstable medical conditions in whom the risk of urgent surgery outweighs the risk of delay. Such patients include those with arrhythmia, acute coronary syndromes, cerebrovascular accidents, sepsis and severe hypoxia. The general consensus appears to suggest that their medical status should be stable and optimal, and they should be re-hydrated appropriately. Patients might not have had anything to drink for hours or even days. They are monitored carefully while being prepared for surgical intervention, which, if possible, should be performed within 24 hours after admission. Fractures may be repaired by screws, pin and plate or a prosthetic femoral head may be inserted with or without cement and intra-operative X-ray imaging may be used.

Spinal anaesthesia is usually chosen because it provides rapid anaesthesia. The short-term mortality is considerably less. However, performing a spinal anaesthesia on a patient with a fracture who is in pain may be very difficult. Hypotension may result. The use of low-volume hyperbaric bupivacaine in sitting position with a fast running intravenous line is helpful. Vasopressors may be required. If general anaesthesia is selected, the dose of drugs must be reduced, intubation of trachea and ventilation method are usually preferred. A laryngeal mask airway is increasingly used but may pose a problem in edentulous patients.

Dislocation of a prosthetic hip needs urgent manipulation to relieve pain. A brief anaesthetic requiring adequate relaxation of muscles may be required.

7.4.2 **Surgery for other fractures**

Other orthopaedic surgery includes fracture of humerus, tibia, fibula, ankle, wrist and others. The use of regional anaesthesia is favoured which include brachial plexus block, peripheral nerve block, intravenous regional anaesthesia and so on. If general anaesthesia is required, a simple anaesthetic technique using a laryngeal mask airway or endotracheal intubation and ventilation may be required. At the end of many procedures, a plaster of Paris cast is applied.

7.5 **Sedation during regional anaesthesia**

Sedation is often used in patients undergoing regional anaesthesia because of the noise arising from the use of instruments during surgery (see Box 7.2). The duration of surgery combined with operative noise as well as the lateral position for hip surgery makes patients restless and uncomfortable. Midazolam titrated in 1 mg aliquots is often used but can occasionally cause confusion and, in excess doses, can lead to loss of control of the airway. However, there are reports of increased morbidity after sedation in elderly and these patients must be monitored carefully.

Box 7.2 Sedation in the elderly

- There is excessive noise during surgery.
- Patient cannot remain in lateral position for a long duration during surgery.
- Sedation is common during regional anaesthesia.
- There are reports of increased morbidity after sedation in elderly.
  - Excess dose of sedative can also lead to loss of control of airway and confusion.

Box 7.3 Thromboembolic prophylaxis in the elderly during major orthopaedic surgery

- DVT is associated particularly with surgery on the pelvis, hip or knee.
- Most DVT episodes occur in the first week after a hip fracture and can lead to PE.
  - Risk is substantial preoperatively or intra-operatively (4–14%).
- There is no universal method of preventing DVT or PE.
- Multiple measures are adopted.
  - Heparin is known to reduce fatal PE in susceptible patients.

7.6 **Thromboembolic prophylaxis**

Although deep vein thrombosis (DVT) may complicate any surgery, it is associated particularly with surgery on the pelvis, hip or knee. DVT prophylaxis is clearly necessary in patients undergoing hip surgery (see Box 7.3). Most DVT episodes occur in the first week after a hip fracture, and the risk is substantial either pre-operatively or intra-operatively. Patients with hip fracture have a high risk of fatal pulmonary embolus (PE), with rates of 4–14%. PE is often fatal in this age group and is the cause for majority of deaths after hip replacement. There is no universal method of preventing DVT and PE and multiple measures are adopted. Heparin is known to reduce fatal PE in susceptible patients. Various studies have compared results of DVT prophylaxis in elderly patients with hip fracture; and although no particular treatment is distinctly superior, some type of medication should be used (warfarin, low-molecular-weight heparin, unfractionated heparin, aspirin, sequential compression devices).

Summaries of the literature suggest that low-molecular-weight heparin (LMWH) may decrease the incidence of DVT more effectively than other therapies; however, this is disputed as the most cost-effective choice. LMWH inhibits the coagulation enzyme Xa and binds antithrombin 3. Managing such therapy and the risks of potent anticoagulation regimens in frail, elderly patients is often difficult. In the setting of selected high-risk patients, aspirin or even simple mechanical measures such as pneumatic compression devices may be effective. Compression stockings have an additive thromboprophylactic benefit with negligible risk and therefore should be used in combination with other treatment.

Evidence supports the use of a therapeutic regimen beginning at the time of hospitalization (pre-operatively). Aspirin or warfarin may be given the night before or after surgery and continued post-operatively per normal dosing regimens. LMWH should not be administered at an interval closer than 12 hours pre-operatively. The available data on the appropriate duration of DVT prophylaxis post-operatively are scarce. At a minimum, patients should continue with at least a daily dose of aspirin and wear compression stockings for 6 weeks post-operatively.

7.7 **Antibiotic prophylaxis**

Orthopaedic surgery is often performed under a laminar flow hood, which blows clean filtered air downwards. Antibiotics are routinely used peri-operatively to decrease the incidence of wound infection in orthopaedic surgery (see Box 7.4). In patients with hip fractures, it is critically important to provide such prophylactic coverage peri-operatively because the integrity of the prosthetic components must also be considered. If drug allergy is not an issue, first or second generation cephalosporins are the antibiotics of choice for the prevention of these infections. Optimal infection prophylaxis is provided by administering the first dose of intravenous antibiotic in the immediate pre-operative period and continuing for a total duration of 24 hours.

Box 7.4 Prevention of infection

- Orthopaedic surgery is often performed under a laminar flow hood.
- Pre-operative use of antibiotics is common.
  - Must be administered before a tourniquet is inflated.
  - Must be continued in the post-operative period.
- Many orthopaedic surgeons insist on the use of face mask.

> **Box 7.5 Temperature control during surgery**
>
> - Hypothermia is common in elderly.
>   - Little subcutaneous fat hence poor insulation.
>   - Transfer of the patient into the cold environment.
>   - Prolonged stay in the anaesthetic room at lower temperature.
>   - Evaporative loss heat from body and operative site during prolonged surgery.
>   - Administration of cold intravenous fluid and blood.
> - Return of core temperature takes longer particularly due to vasodilatation after central neuro-axial block.
> - Hypothermia is associated with increased risk of infection.
> - Measures should be taken to prevent hypothermia by using forced air warming system, by heating intravenous fluid/blood and by utilising impermeable surgical drapes.

7.8 **Temperature imbalance**

Heat is redistributed from core to periphery during anaesthesia, leading to reduced body temperature (see Box 7.5). Hypothermia is often present on transfer from the ward and active warming should be considered, especially if a prolonged period in the anaesthetic room is envisaged. There is very little subcutaneous fat in the elderly for insulation and evaporative loss from the body and operative site may be excessive. Intravenous fluid stored at room temperature if not administered through a blood warmer will further decrease body temperature. Return of core temperature takes longer especially after the vasodilatation due to central neuro-axial block. Hypothermia is known to be associated with increased blood loss and risk of infection. Intra-operatively the most effective way of maintaining normothermia is by forced air warming system, by administering heating intravenous fluid and by utilising impermeable surgical drapes.

7.9 **Blood loss**

Blood loss may be extensive during revision hip surgery and towards the end of knee surgery following the release of tourniquet. Some blood is lost into the deeper tissues. Blood loss can be minimized by maintaining normothermia, good surgical technique and positioning the patient. Epidural and spinal anaesthesia also help to reduce blood loss.

If excessive blood loss is anticipated, pre-deposit donation of blood by the patient and acute normovolaemic haemodilution may help. Drugs which increase bleeding such as non-steroidal anti-inflammatory drugs (NSAIDs) and aspirin should be stopped well in advance.

7.10 **Post-operative pain relief**

Post-operative pain after orthopaedic surgery is usually short-lived but some operations, such as knee surgery, are very painful. Effective pain relief helps in mobilization. A regional technique with opioids provides good and prolonged pain relief. Epidural analgesia with potent local anaesthetic agents may cause prolonged motor block which will hinder mobilization. Hypotension, respiratory depression and urinary retention may also occur with epidural block. Continuous infusions through peripheral catheters or infiltration of local anaesthetic may provide useful analgesia. PCA with an intravenous opioid is a good method of pain relief but some elderly may not use it properly because of arthritis or impaired cognitive function. For both hip and knee surgery, the regular use of paracetamol, other NSAIDs, and weak opioids for moderate or low-intensity pain is recommended for continuing analgesia after the primary analgesic techniques for high intensity pain have worn off or been discontinued.

7.11 **Urinary retention**

Urinary bladder catheter may be required in many patients because of the need for immobilization before or after surgery. Prolonged use of an indwelling urinary catheter is associated with an increased risk of urinary retention and infection. Catheters should routinely be removed when patients are able to get out of bed. If urinary retention occurs after removal of the catheter, intermittent catheterisation should be used to maintain low bladder volumes and decrease the risk of infection.

7.12 **Impaired cognitive function**

Delirium is a common problem in elderly hospitalized patients and occurs to some degree in the vast majority of patients with other dysfunction (see also Chapters 5 and 13). The most important risk factors for delirium are advanced age, dementia, alcohol use and pre-hospitalization functional status. Drugs such as opioids, sedative-hypnotics, anticholinergics and anticonvulsants may predispose to this condition. Fat embolism can be a major cause of delirium and even death in a patient with hip fracture. Other important and frequently encountered causative factors include urinary retention, uncontrolled pain, medications used for pain and the change in environment from home to hospital.

If delirium does occur, the patient should be carefully evaluated for an underlying cause. After surgery the cause is usually multifactorial. The most common contributing yet treatable causes include hypoxia, infection, fluid and electrolyte abnormalities, drug toxicity and hypotension. Excellent geriatric nursing care with reassurance, reorientation and provision of adequate pain control is essential. In addition, environmental adjustments should be made to help prevent sleep deprivation.

7.13 **Rehabilitation and recovery**

Early mobilization and ambulation within 24 hours of surgery is standard practice. Studies have shown that this strategy is safe for most patients and that it is associated with a trend toward earlier discharge. There also may be long-term benefits in functional status. During rehabilitation, a patient's risk of falling should be carefully assessed. Gait training and exercise programs are effective in reducing the long-term risk of subsequent falls. Most hip fractures in elderly patients occur due to osteoporosis. During the recovery process, treatment for osteoporosis is addressed when appropriate. Medical regimens should be reviewed for use of calcium and vitamin D, bisphosphonates or calcitonin should be considered. Estrogen therapy should be reserved until after convalescence because of its known thrombogenic potential. A plan for follow-up and re-evaluation should be established before a patient is discharged. If bone densitometry is used to evaluate the response to therapy, an outpatient baseline study should be obtained.

Further reading

Curran J. Anaesthesia for orthopaedic surgery. In *Textbook of Anaesthesia*, Aitkinhead AR, Rowbotham DJ and Smith Graham, Eds. 4th edition, 2001, Churchill Livingstone, Edinburgh, pp. 582–589.

Gordon HV and Murphy FL. Anesthesia for orthopaedic surgery. In *Wyeli and Curchil Davidson's A Practice of Anaesthesia*, Healy TJ and Knight PR, Eds. 7th edition, 2003, Arnold, London, pp. 707–718.

Horlocker TT, Wedel DJ. Anesthesia for orthopaedic surgery. In *Clinical Anesthesia*, Barash PG, Cullen BF and Stoelting RK, Eds. 5th edition, 2006, Lippincott Williams & Wilkins, Philadelphia, pp. 1112–1128.

Sharrock NE, Beckman JD, Inda EC and Savrese JJ. Anesthesia for orthopaedic surgery. In *Miller's Anesthesia*, Millar RD, Ed. 6th edition, 2005, Elsevier Churchill Livingstone, Philadelphia, pp. 2409–2434.

Chapter 8

Anaesthesia for major abdominal surgery in the elderly

Key points

- Emergency abdominal surgery is the highest risk for mortality in the elderly.
- Assessment of dehydration is imperative.
- Direct (intra-arterial) monitoring of blood pressure is necessary.
- Effective analgesia improves outcome.
- Only experienced anaesthetists should manage emergency abdominal surgical cases.
- Not all abdominal pain is surgically treatable.
- Fluid losses are very common and may be difficult to measure.
- Temperature loss is universal.
- Nitrous oxide causes bowel distension and should be avoided.

Demographic studies show that the numbers of 'old olds' (75–84 years) and 'oldest' (85+) people are increasing in our population. This trend is projected to continue with an estimated 3.8% of the population being in the 'old old' group by 2031. Consequently an increasing number of elderly patients will present for elective as well as emergency surgery. The preparation for elective surgery, which requires an assessment of functional reserve as well as planning for post-operative care, is necessarily restricted in the emergency setting. Unfortunately, these emergency patients are also the most severely compromised ones who most need careful but rapid resuscitation prior to surgery. The preparation and management of these patients are described for elective surgery and key areas highlighted for the emergency cases later.

The normal process of ageing results in a number of pathophysiological changes, which influence an individual's responses to anaesthesia and surgery (see Chapter 2). In addition many of these patients may have associated, possibly advanced, co-morbidities. These factors need to be taken into consideration before embarking on anaesthesia for major abdominal surgery in elderly patients.

Although basal physiological function may often be well preserved with increasing age, the elderly show a progressive decline in functional reserve limiting their ability to cope with the stress of anaesthesia and surgery. The pharmacokinetic properties and pharmacodynamic effects of some drugs may be different in the elderly with changes in volume of distribution, metabolism and elimination (see Chapter 3).

As a consequence, the elderly patient may already be receiving a variety of drug therapies with an increased potential for drug errors and interactions. Compliance is often poor prior to admission and several drugs may need to be stopped before surgery, while the continuation of others remains essential. The elderly may have compromised nutritional status. Cognitive impairment, loss of visual and hearing acuity may compromise peri-operative management.

A number of factors have been associated with or identified as risk factors for deterioration post-operatively in elderly patients, particularly with regard to post-operative delirium and post-operative cognitive dysfunction (see Chapter 13). These include age, pre-operative dementia and depression, intra-operative blood loss, post-operative anaemia, anticholinergic drug administration and pain.

8.1 **Elective abdominal surgery**

8.1.1 **Surgical preparation**

Many surgical procedures involve the colon and rectum and are preceded by, often vigorous, bowel preparation. This usually involves the administration of potent laxatives and enemata to clear as much faecal matter as possible. Unfortunately, they also cause marked water loss. This is frequently severe enough to lead to dehydration (Table 8.1) that necessitates treatment prior to surgery. The patient should be weighed prior to bowel preparation and regularly before surgery. All weight loss can be assumed to be fluid loss and should be replaced, volume by volume, with a physiological saline solution.

8.1.2 **Pre-medication**

Many elderly patients are very anxious and frightened in a strange environment. They may have a short-term memory loss and, despite explanations, many are completely unaware of what is going to happen to them. It used to be good practice to prescribe benzodiazepines to allay this anxiety, but the duration of action of benzodiazepines can be

Table 8.1 Severity and signs of dehydration			
Severity	Body weight loss (%)	Estimated volume loss (L)	Clinical signs
Mild	4	3	Thirst (unreliable in the elderly) dry mucous membranes Capillary refill time >2 seconds Skin turgor reduced (unreliable in the elderly)
Moderate	5–8	4–6	All above + Tachycardia Oliguria (<0.5 ml kg^{-1} h^{-1}) Postural hypotension
Severe	8-10	7+	All above + Hypotension Imminent cardiovascular collapse

very prolonged in the elderly. This is less pronounced with temazepam than diazepam but because of these concerns pre-medication is generally avoided.

8.1.3 **Monitoring**

Standard patient monitoring should be instituted upon entering the anaesthetic room. Unless there are contraindications, invasive monitoring should be instituted prior to induction. The beat-to-beat real-time information obtained from invasive monitoring of arterial blood pressure may be beneficial in high-risk patients. Atrial fibrillation, common in the elderly, may render automated non-invasive blood pressure monitoring inaccurate and is prone to delay due to the beat-to-beat variation in pulse pressure. Arterial access also allows near patient testing of haemoglobin concentration and acid–base status. Central venous pressure monitoring is mostly accessed via the internal jugular vein, while the use of a long-line sited in the antecubital fossa is an alternative less-invasive approach. Monitoring of neuromuscular function and temperature are equally important.

8.1.4 **Choice of intravenous induction agent**

The initial distribution of drug is often impaired in elderly. Protein binding is less efficient. Induction agents should be administered more slowly, and with longer pauses between bolus doses than in the younger patient because prolongation of arm–brain circulation time increases the time taken for the patient to lose consciousness. Reduced protein binding coupled with a contracted blood volume lead to a higher free drug concentration. An overdose may easily occur, which will lead to inadvertent marked cardiorespiratory side effects. The haemodynamic consequences of propofol induction are enhanced and delayed in the elderly. Etomidate may have advantages due to its improved cardiovascular stability, particularly in patients in whom there is considerable cardiac compromise as there are concerns of adrenal suppression following administration of even a single dose. The incidence of side effects is similar with propofol and thiopentone. The use of short acting opioids such as fentanyl or alfentanil reduces the dose of induction agent required and attenuates the stress response to laryngoscopy.

8.1.5 Choice of inhalational anaesthetic agents

The minimum alveolar concentration (MAC) of all inhalational anaesthetic agents is reduced by 20–40% from young adult values. Desflurane may allow earlier extubation particularly after prolonged surgery; however the earlier recovery characteristics compared with other agents are short-lived. Sevoflurane has been used extensively in the elderly because it is relatively non-irritant for both induction and maintenance of anaesthesia and appears to be an attractive option because of relatively fewer cardiovascular side effects. Gas induction is likely to be slower in the elderly due to ventilation/perfusion mismatch which can be exacerbated by the elderly supine patient having their closing capacity within tidal breathing. An air–oxygen mixture is preferred as a carrier gas rather than nitrous oxide (to avoid bowel distension and increased incidence of nausea and vomitting).

8.1.6 Choice of analgesic agents

Opioid pharmacokinetics is hardly affected by age but central nervous system sensitivity to these drugs is markedly increased in the elderly. The dose of opioids should be reduced in the elderly. However, there are marked inter-individual variations. Remifentanil appears to be a better drug because of its titrability and absence of lingering effect however the dose must be titrated carefully. Haemodynamic depression is known to occur with excessive doses.

8.1.7 Choice of neuromuscular blocking agents

Ageing is associated with a reduction in muscle mass, which may be expected to lower the dose requirement of neuromuscular blocking drugs. However, the potency of neuromuscular blocking drugs is similar in all adult populations owing to the development of extra-junctional cholinergic receptors in the elderly. Depolarising muscle relaxant is generally avoided in elective patients unless their use is warranted (prevention of acid aspiration). Vecuronium and rocuronuim demonstrate a slower onset and longer duration of action than in younger patients when compared with atracuruim and cisatracuruim. Atracurium is the preferred drug as its duration of action is very similar to that in younger patients. Hoffman degradation and spontaneous ester hydrolysis compensates for the reduction in hepatic clearance.

Dose requirements of neuromuscular blocking agent for maintenance are reduced by concurrent use of other anaesthetic agents used during anaesthesia. Reversal of neuromuscular blockade with anticholinesterase drugs tends to be similar to that in younger adults, with less increase in heart rate from the accompanying anticholinergic. Monitoring of neuromuscular functions is highly desirable.

8.1.8 Airway maintenance

Intubation and controlled ventilation are the preferred choices during major abdominal surgery. Muscle relaxation is required to secure the airway, although care needs to be taken in securing the endotracheal tube, as adhesive tape may damage the frail skin in elderly. Intubation is sometimes difficult in patients with arthritis who have reduced neck mobility but generally these patients are edentulous. The obtunded protective airway reflexes, reduction in gastric emptying and reduced gastro-oesophageal sphincter tone all make reflux of gastric contents and subsequent aspiration more likely in the elderly. The use of narrower endotracheal tubes reduces the incidence of sore throat in the post-operative period. Normal levels of oxygenation and normocapnia should be maintained. Ventilation pressures should be kept as low as possible. The addition of slight positive end-expiratory pressure (PEEP) may be required to maintain haemoglobin saturation.

8.1.9 Intravenous fluid administration

The aim of fluid management peri-operatively is to maintain hydration, electrolyte homeostasis, haemodynamic stability, organ perfusion and function. Urinary losses as well as third space loss, fluid sequestration into the gut and loss from high-output stoma sites all need to be considered in terms of fluid and electrolyte therapy. Loss of potassium, chloride, magnesium and phosphate together with malabsorption may all be issues in the peri-operative and post-operative periods. Large bore intravenous access will be required unless for minor surgery but securing intravenous cannulae may be difficult due to skin fragility. Care needs to be taken if fluids are administered under pressure, as fragile vessel walls may rupture leading to extravasations of fluids. Hypovolaemia is a major contributor to hypotension during the peri-operative and post-operative periods. The elderly are less able to compensate for hypovolaemia due to the effects of ageing on cardiovascular and renal systems.

A urinary catheter should be used throughout the peri-operative period, although the presence of a urine output may only indicate an adequate rather than optimum fluid balance. Central venous pressure monitoring may be beneficial in the elderly, but may not be a reliable guide to fluid status. A worsening base deficit from arterial blood gas analysis may imply that organ perfusion is compromised due to hypovolaemia. Patient positioning may have an impact on the adequacy of fluid replacement. The increase in venous return seen when the patient is placed in the head-down position may falsely elevate central venous and arterial blood pressures resulting in reduced fluid replacement unless these postural changes are taken into consideration. The use of oesophageal Doppler as a less-invasive way of monitoring cardiac output to direct fluid replacement has received attention and appears to offer benefits over conventional invasive monitoring.

Blood loss may vary with the type of surgery. Blood loss is often insidious with little measured blood loss in suction containers. Swabs should be weighed throughout surgery in order to obtain accurate estimates of blood loss. Blood replacement is better instituted using transfusion triggers based on near patient testing of haemoglobin or haematocrit. Although a haemoglobin concentration of 7–8 g dL^{-1} may be well tolerated in the younger population, this may be less acceptable in the elderly owing to the presence of cardiac disease and reduced cardiac reserve. Blood transfusion should always be considered if there is excessive blood loss.

8.1.10 **Temperature maintenance**

Maintenance of body temperature is essential during the peri-operative period, and should start when the patient enters the theatre environment. Hypothermia is more common in the elderly, and these patients are less able to conserve body temperature due to the effects of ageing. Although they have reduced muscle bulk that reduces the oxygen demand created by shivering, this may still impose a requirement that exceeds respiratory and cardiac reserve, although the effects may not be as great as once thought. Elderly patients also lack the metabolic and muscular reserve to restore their body temperature back to normal levels. There is a tendency for body temperature to fall during anaesthesia (poikilothermia) due to vasodilation and a distribution of blood away from the core, lack of thermoregulatory control and loss of heat to the environment. Hypothermia is associated with an increase in wound infection, delayed removal of sutures and prolonged hospital stay.

Patients will frequently be hypothermic by the time they enter theatre from the anaesthetic room, particularly if the anaesthetic time is prolonged from establishing an epidural and inserting invasive monitoring. Further evaporative heat losses occur from the exposed surgical site, and it may be difficult to restore normothermia unless all available measures are used. Passive measures such as reflective drapes and warmed intravenous fluids can only help prevent heat loss. The use of epidural anaesthesia during the peri-operative period means that heat loss from the lower extremities is increased due to sympathetically mediated vasodilatation. In order to restore a hypothermic patient to normothermia, forced warm air systems and warming mattresses are more useful, particularly if placed on the lower extremities. However patient positioning, particularly the Lloyd–Davis position, means that it can be difficult to utilize all these methods. Core temperature monitoring is easily achieved with naso-pharyngeal temperature probes. The core temperature should be within normal limits before the patient leaves the recovery area.

8.1.11 **Positioning**

Positioning may pose a challenge owing to the reduced joint mobility from arthritic changes or previous prosthetic joint replacement. The supine position is usually not a problem but surgery may be done in the Lloyd–Davis, left lateral or prone jack-knife positions. Care should be taken to ensure that pressure areas are well padded to avoid nerve injury and pressure sores. The latter may be debilitating and entail a hospital stay longer than that for the original surgery.

8.1.12 **Post-operative pain control**

A mid-line incision is common during major abdominal surgery and this is associated with significant pain because the incision crosses several dermatomes. More surgery is being performed with trans-verse or muscle splitting incisions to reduce the impact of a mid-line incision on respiratory function as well as for the reduction in pain.

Pain is not only unpleasant but it can also contribute to potential morbidity and mortality. Pain can affect every organ system and this includes impaired respiratory function as deep breathing exacerbates the pain; the patient therefore avoids this and fails to expand their lung bases. This effect is believed to lead to the retention of respira-tory tract secretions and an increase in the incidence of pneumonia and respiratory failure. Haemodynamic changes can occur as the pain results in an enhanced stress response, tachycardia and hypertension. Patients undergoing abdominal surgery will require significant levels of peri-operative and post-operative analgesia.

Peri-operatively, analgesia options include morphine, remifentanil infusion or epidural analgesia. Post-operative pain control is most easily achieved with patient controlled epidural analgesia (PCEA) or patient controlled analgesia (PCA) using morphine. However the presence of confusion and cognitive dysfunction may make assess-ment of pain and treatment with PCEA/PCA techniques problematic.

The evidence supporting the claim that epidural analgesia is associated with improved outcomes is not very clear but reduced respiratory complications and thrombotic complications have been demonstrated. Epidural analgesia may offer better quality post-operative analgesia than other regimens, however there is little evidence from trials carried out exclusively in the elderly. Epidural analgesia may be asso-ciated with a significant failure rate unless intensive and active follow-up is implemented. The epidural should ideally be inserted in the awake patient. The catheter should be sited at the appropriate level for surgery while minimising the risk of spinal cord damage. For abdominal surgery, the catheter is most appropriately placed at lower thoracic spaces (T8–T11). The use of low-dose local anaesthetic combined with low-dose opioid is commonly used. The use of higher strength solutions of local anaesthetic agent such as 0.5% bupivacaine are more likely to be associated with motor weakness and a greater drop in blood pressure, depending on the degree of sympathetic blockade produced. Patients are usually more awake, mobile and suffer less nausea and vomiting compared with those in which intravenous opiate is used. It is essential that the patient is nursed in an area where the staff is familiar with epidurals and their complications, and have the time and expertise to look after the patient.

Alternatively intravenous morphine is administered through a PCA machine using a bolus regimen with a set lock-out interval. Analgesia is first achieved with intermittent titrated loading dose of morphine and then a PCA machine is attached. However, the use of a background infusion should be avoided as it is associated with an increased incidence of hypoxia and respiratory depression. Other side effects include nausea, vomiting, dreams, hallucinations, temporary impairment of cognitive function and others.

Non-steroidal anti-inflammatory drugs (NSAIDS) are useful adjuncts to both PCEA and PCA. However, the benefits need to be balanced against the risk of renal complications caused by using these drugs in patients with pre-existing age-related renal dysfunction, impaired fluid handling and the potential for post-operative hypovolaemia. The choice of analgesic technique should weigh up all risks and benefits including patient preference.

8.1.13 **Post-operative oxygen administration**

Oxygen is administered to prevent post-operative hypoxaemia and myocardial ischaemia. High concentrations of oxygen have been associated with a decreased incidence of wound infection and post-operative nausea and vomiting; therefore, it seems appropriate to use a high level of oxygen intra-operatively and in the recovery phase.

8.1.14 **Post-operative care**

The elderly patients should receive post-operative care in an environment that is appropriate to the degree of co-morbidity and type of surgery. They are more likely to require high dependency or intensive care facilities post-operatively. A high patient/nurse ratio allows closer attention to oxygenation, fluid balance, acid–base status and analgesia and recognition of post-operative complications may be noted sooner. Chest physiotherapy and incentive spirometry may also be appropriate. Early mobilization should be encouraged. The patient should receive continuous humidified oxygen particularly while epidural or PCA opiates are being used. Epidural analgesia is usually continued for 3–5 days, supplemented by simple oral analgesics such as paracetamol.

The elderly patient presenting for abdominal surgery presents a significant challenge. This group of patients undergoing intra-abdominal surgery is considered to be in one of the highest risk groups for cardiac complications. They should be managed by health care professionals who are aware of the needs of elderly and appropriately tailor the anaesthetic and the surgery accordingly.

8.2 Anaesthesia for emergency abdominal surgery

This is the most common life-threatening surgical presentation in the elderly. It carries a high mortality and morbidity and should only be managed by experienced anaesthetists. All the considerations discussed above are necessary, but the time to assess, resuscitate and present to theatre is short and when urgent will occur concurrently. A critical review of the non-surgical causes of acute abdominal pain, inferior myocardial infarction, pancreatitis, ketoacidosis or porphyria, for instance, should be performed.

Emergency surgery is often carried out for obstruction, gastro-intestinal bleeding or peritonitis. The diagnosis may not be known and the duration of surgery may be unduly prolonged. Pain relief should be started before surgery as should fluid replacement therapy. Abdominal distension from the ileus should be treated with aspiration through a naso-gastric tube, and this should be left on free drainage throughout.

A rapid sequence induction is indicated. Although basic principles and practice of anaesthesia is essentially similar to elective procedures, one has to be prepared for all potential complications, including vomiting and regurgitation, hypovolaemia, haemorrhage, cardiovascular disturbances, abnormal reaction to drugs in the presence of electrolytes disturbances and probably renal impairment (see Chapter 6). Complete cardiovascular and other monitoring may be required.

Provision of post-operative pain relief and post-operative care are especially important as there are usually percutaneous drains in situ and these increase the pain especially on movement. Pain assessment in the elderly is poor and requires a dedicated carer to assess this regularly and ensure that effective analgesia is both prescribed and administered. These patients usually receive intravenous opiate through a PCA machine as there may not be time for epidural anaesthesia and in certain cases may not be appropriate.

The impact of an acute surgical procedure for an abdominal emergency will challenge the organ function of renal, hepatic and immunological systems. Post-operative complications should be expected in all organ systems, and these patients are likely to require nursing and medical care in a critical care bed area requiring attention of experienced clinicians.

Further reading

Anaesthesia and Peri-Operative Care of the Elderly. The Association of Anaesthetists of Great Britain and Ireland, London, December 2001 (http://www.aagbi.org/publications/htm, website accessed on 3rd June 2007).

Aubrun F. Management of postoperative analgesia in elderly patients. *Reg Anesth Pain Med* 2005; **30**: 363–380.

Cook DJ and Rooke GA. Priorities in perioperative geriatrics. *Anesth Analg* 2003; **96**: 1823–1836.

Nimmo SM. Rapid recovery after major abdominal surgery. In *Gastrointestinal and Colorectal Anesthesia*. Kumar and Bellamy Eds. Informa healthcare 2006.

Chapter 9

Neurosurgery in the elderly

> **Key points**
> - Neurosurgical procedures are commonly performed in the elderly.
> - Palliative procedures are more common in the elderly.
> - Degenerative conditions are more likely to present for surgical treatment in the elderly.
> - Spinal cord blood supply is often compromised.
> - There are no fast neurosurgical operations.
> - Temperature loss can be significant.
> - Positioning may be difficult.
> - Pressure sores, deep vein thrombosis (DVT) and nerve damage are more likely to occur.
> - Remifentanil and desflurane are particularly valuable in the elderly neurosurgical patient.

Until the later years of the twentieth century, the belief remained that neurosurgical procedures on the elderly were associated with poor outcomes. The development of surgical techniques and anaesthesia has mitigated this position and many more procedures are now performed on these patients.

These operations largely fall into two groups:

1. Operations that are now being performed in older groups although they have been available to younger patients for some time.
2. New operations that have an age-related bias.

The former range from surgery for intracranial tumours to spinal procedures to relieve cord compression while the latter include aggressive surgery for pain relief and palliation following malignant vertebral collapse. These procedures can be further divided into those that are related to the axial skeleton/cranio-cervical junction and intracranial procedures.

9.1 Anaesthetic considerations

Most neurosurgical procedures are relatively urgent. This may be immediate if there is a grossly raised intracranial pressure or sudden onset of cord compression. Most can be managed within a week of presentation and some are truly elective. Prior activity levels and cognitive function are essential elements in the pre-anaesthetic screening because they will determine outcome and therefore the choice of operation and anaesthetic technique.

Most neurosurgical operations take at least an hour and many last 4–7 hours. It is not uncommon for reconstructive surgery to take more than 10 hours. Although these pose problems in young fit patients, they may be insurmountable for the elderly. It is rare that complete recovery occurs after neurosurgery, unless the operation involves 'silent' areas of the brain.

Concurrent drug therapy has to be reviewed and decisions about continuing this medication for the peri-operative period have to be made. Most drugs do not have a severe withdrawal effect but alcohol and nicotine do. Many patients are started on steroids to reduce tumour size and these can precipitate a diabetic state especially in the elderly.

There are several aspects of anaesthesia that are important and worth re-emphasising.

For patients, there are many emergency operations in which either the brain or the spinal cord function is at risk from a reduced perfusion pressure. This may be due to increased fluid (oedema), due to neuronal damage, from hypotension or from hypoxia for example. There are several strategies to try to manage this but they differ between brain and spinal cord.

Hyperventilation is the most common technique used to try to acutely lower intracranial pressure and improve cerebral perfusion pressure. The relationship between arterial carbon dioxide concentrations and cerebral vasoconstriction is maintained with age, but the elderly brain tolerates falls in metabolic substrate delivery poorly. The mean blood flow to the brain does fall with advancing age but this probably reflects the cellular neuronal loss that also occurs (Figure 9.1).

There is little data on the impact of hyperventilation on the management of cord ischaemia secondary to increased spinal canal pressure, although increasing ventilation to reduce arterial carbon dioxide concentrations will increase the mean intra-thoracic and potentially indirectly increase the transmitted pressure into the thoracic spinal canal. A reduction in inferior vena cava return and epidural diversion of venous return is another possible unintended consequence of hyperventilation.

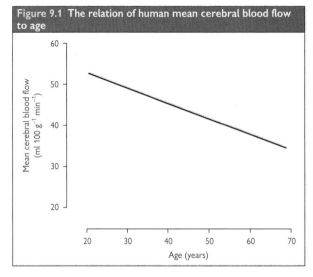

Figure 9.1 **The relation of human mean cerebral blood flow to age**

Temperature control in the elderly is more fragile than in younger patients. This is partly due to a fall in metabolic rate and ability to shiver, but a proportion of elderly patients have disordered central thermostatic control. They are more prone to hypothermia in all environments including operation theatres and wards. The evidence on wound infection rates and sepsis related to mild hypothermia suggest that aggressive prevention is necessary from arrival in the theatre complex to discharge to the post-operative ward.

Availability of anaesthetic agents has changed over the recent years and two of them in particular have made care of the elderly more precise. These are remifentanil and desflurane.

Remifentanil because of its plasma esterase elimination has similar properties across the range of ages. Its rapid onset and offset that is largely time independent allows profound pain relief and respiratory drive suppression peri-operatively with a smooth and swift return to normal. This allows active management of recovery from anaesthesia and controlled return of consciousness without coughing on the endotracheal tube. This is invaluable after surgery for intracranial haemorrhage or clot removal.

Desflurane is highly lipid insoluble, more so than sevoflurane, and this is very advantageous in the elderly because they have a greater proportion of their body mass as fat than do younger patients of the same body mass index. Recovery profiles are little affected by age

Permission to reproduce Figure 9.1 sought from Dr Harold T. Davenport.

and duration of administration. When combined with remifentanil, recovery can be managed and there is a choice between awake but non-coughing recovery and full return of effective ventilation before arousal.

Intramuscular administration should be avoided in the elderly because they are no longer the 'vessel-rich' group seen in younger patients and plasma drug concentrations are therefore very unpredictable. Equally they predispose to pressure sore development and contractures because of the delayed absorption of high concentrations of drug from the muscle bodies. For these reasons intravenous or oral opiates and non-steroidal anti-inflammatory drugs are preferred.

9.2 **Spinal surgery**

Increasingly, degenerative diseases affecting the vertebral column such as severe rheumatoid arthrosis, osteoporosis or osteoarthrosis are being treated by instrumental decompression and fixation irrespective of the age of the patient. This is because their results in terms of retained function nearly match those of younger patients.

The key determinants of successful outcome depend on the careful assessment of pre-existing function and the impact that any myelopathy has on daily activities. It is unusual for these to improve following surgery, as the primary aim is to prevent further deterioration. Assessment of pulmonary function is arguably the most important factor in recovery.

However, there are specific problems related to the changes in vascular structure and neuronal function with advancing age. The blood supply to the spinal cord is by one anterior and two pairs of posterior arteries that descend through the foramen magnum and course to the lower end of the cord. But below the 'watershed' at T4/5, perfusion is more dependent on fine feeding arteries from the descending aorta and these become more tortuous and rigid with increasing age. Kinking of these vessels during operative positioning or surgical traction can lead to unexpected cord ischaemia during apparently routine operations. The spinal perfusion pressure is analogous to the cerebral perfusion pressure and is largely determined by the pressure within the spinal canal and the mean arterial pressure. Hypotensive episodes can be predictably harmful if there is a raised pressure within the spinal canal, for instance from a tumour or vertebral collapse.

In general, neurosurgical procedures take a long time and this time increases if there is a need for instrumentation and fixation following cord decompression. Elderly soft tissues are more friable and less supportive than that of younger patients and they have more osteophytic changes in their spinal column. This can make surgical positioning and access difficult. Pressure sores are a high risk and all precautions must be used to try to prevent this life-threatening complication.

9.2.1 Specific operations

9.2.1.1 Cervical and lumbar discectomy

Decompression procedures usually involve removal of disc material as in younger patients. This may be as an urgent procedure if the cord is acutely compressed, or more usually, an elective one where segmental neuronal symptoms are present. The differences lie in the ability to position an elderly spine especially if a frame is necessary for support in the prone position. The elderly are more likely to become hypotensive on lying prone and the increased intraocular pressure in this position increases the risk of retinal as well as corneal damage.

In common with all patient transfers in the elderly, rolling and sliding may cause intense pain in the manipulated joints, which can be more severe than the site of incision.

The anterior approach to the cervical cord may be difficult because of the limited movements of the cervical spine with increasing age. Ligaments are less robust and osteophytes may obscure the normal bony landmarks. Rigid vessels will bleed more once damaged and it is more difficult to achieve haemostasis. The risk to the cervical cord of slipping off the bone when drilling off these hard osteophytes is ever present.

Pain is rarely a problem, but post-operative vigilance is necessary where the operative level is above the larynx because of the risk of post-operative oedema or bleeding. A drain is mandatory.

Odontoid decompression is warranted in patients with severe rheumatoid disease where there is a progressive laxity of the longitudinal ligaments. This leads to brain stem, medulla or cord compression by the odontoid and there are symptoms of a high cord lesion. The progressive myelopathy that affects the lower and then upper limbs leads to great dependency before restricting pulmonary function and ultimately respiratory failure.

The route of surgical access is trans-oral, with an incision through the soft palate and the lower naso-pharynx. Retraction may lead to glossal oedema, and tissue handling increases the risk of upper airway oedema post-operatively. Securing the airway orally is normal; however some surgeons prefer a nasal endotracheal tube and a large bore naso-gastric tube (which they use to support their retractors). The naso-gastric tube has to remain in situ for several post-operative days until swallowing is back to normal.

Although the procedure is prolonged and usually uneventful, manipulation of the odontoid can directly compress the brain stem with results that range from asystolic vascular collapse to severe tachycardiac hypertension. Drilling through the rheumatoid pannus may expose aberrantly positioned vertebral arteries at the second cervical vertebral level.

Spinal instrumental fusion is increasingly used in primary decompression of the disc spaces because of the superior stability that is achieved and prolonged benefit to the patient. This is also true of more elderly patients, but these are long operations. Blood loss may be greater and a low threshold for replacement transfusion is necessary. Vertebrectomy is an option where there is collapse of a single vertebral body. This is often secondary to metastatic spread of tumour, and the aim of surgery is to prevent further loss of neuromuscular control and prevent or alleviate the associated pain. The vertebral body is exposed and removed, often with major blood loss, and a cage implanted between the adjoining bodies to provide mechanical stability. Bone graft material is used to provide initial stability while healing and fibrosis take place.

Osteoporotic vertebral collapse causes immobility due to the severe pain and muscle spasm. This may last several weeks and can be dramatically improved by vertebroplasty. This usually involves image-guided placement of a large (epidural) 16 g cannula into the vertebral body and then injecting acrylic cement to fix the body. This procedure is almost immediately effective but there have been reports of cardiovascular collapse similar to that seen with cemented hip prosthesis insertion.

9.3 **Intracranial surgery**

Acute/chronic subdural haematoma is a common finding in elderly patients who have had a fall and then become delirious. The decision on whether to evacuate the haematoma in such frail patients is not clear-cut. The pre-injury status of the patient is a vital part of the decision-making process. If they were in a fully dependent environment with disordered cognitive function, little improvement is likely; whereas if they had been independent and very socially active, some optimism would be justified. Re-bleeding is common and sudden changes in their level of consciousness should alert the team that this may have occurred. Rapid rescanning and possibly further drainage must be considered.

9.3.1 **Tumours**

Intracranial tumours are commonly metastatic in the elderly although all other common primary lesions can occur. Presentation may differ in that the progressive loss of brain substance with ageing will limit early signs of a raised intracranial pressure. As the brain is an immunologically isolated site, occasionally a secondary metastasis is found without an identifiable primary. The prognosis in these patients is usually very good.

Unfortunately, the elderly brain poorly tolerates retraction and hypotension. Hyperventilation is rarely needed and is best used for only very short periods when pressure reduction is imperative. As with spinal surgery, positioning can pose problems for the elderly patient, especially if posterior fossa surgery is planned. The sitting position is rarely used in the elderly because of the difficulty in maintaining cardiovascular stability.

There is an increased drive to rapidly assess and treat patients who present with stroke. Many of these are occlusive events and, after rapid clinical evaluation and MRI investigations with contrast to identify areas with critical perfusion, thrombolytic therapy is started. For those patients who have a haemorrhage, surgery is likely to be considered. The reduction in clot size improves the vasospasm commonly present and improves outcome in a similar manner to the thrombolysis. This aggressive surgery is performed at only a few centres currently while outcome data is collected.

Endocrine disease increases in prevalence with ageing and this is reflected in the number of patients who have a pituitary adenoma. These are usually removed trans-nasally. The use of potent vasoconstrictors may be problematic in the elderly because of the potential rise in blood pressure that can accompany their use.

Neurosurgical management of other medical conditions has resurged with the advent of sterotactic guidance systems that allow very accurate positioning of probes within the brain. This has been used to treat the tremor associated with Parkinson's disease and for intractable epilepsy for some time. These procedures usually require a 'wake-up' during the anaesthesia to confirm the correct placement of the probe. The speed and completeness of arousal is reduced in the elderly and greater skills and judgement are required to achieve this. Alternatives using gamma sources have been used with success.

The implantation of stem cells to try to regenerate failed neurological systems have met with little success, largely because the use of mesodermal stem cells in ectodermal cell lines is ill-considered. Recent work has been more promising.

Trigeminal neuralgia is a severely painful condition that may become unresponsive to medication. Lesioning the trigeminal nerve can stop this painful process and such is the intensity of the pain that most patients will accept a major posterior fossa exploration to gain the benefit. Positioning to allow surgical access to the trigeminal fossa can be difficult especially in the elderly.

9.4 **Summary**

The elderly are more likely to undergo neurosurgery than in the past, and many of these procedures are specifically for conditions closely related to ageing. Their responses to anaesthesia and the 'routine' intra-operative techniques such as hypoventilation do differ considerably and great care is needed in their use. Positioning and padding once positioned are more important than in younger patients as their risk of tissue damage, nerve or skin, is that much greater.

Further reading

Aitkenhead AR, Rowbotham DJ, Smith G, Eds. (2001). *Textbook of Anaesthesia*. Churchill Livingstone, ISBN 0443063818: Chapter 57.

Hutton P, Cooper GM, James III FM and Butterworth IV JF, Eds. (2002). *Fundamental Principles and Practice of Anaesthesia*. Martin Dunitz Ltd, UK IABN 1-899066-57-8. Chapter 43 and 63.

Chapter 10

Urological and gynaecological surgery in the elderly

Key points

- The most common urological and gynaecological procedures performed in very old patients are mainly endoscopic or perineal.
- Urinary tract endoscopy and surgery should be performed on sterile urine.
- Simple measures may prevent most of the transurethral resection of the prostate (TURP) syndrome cases.
- Endoscopic urological surgery in patients on chronic anti-platelet treatment may lead to life threatening haemorrhage, but interruption of the anti-platelet drug(s) must be kept to a minimum.
- Modern general anaesthetic techniques may challenge the dominant position of spinal anaesthesia.

10.1 Common urological and gynaecological procedures

Apart from major carcinological procedures which have no specificities in the elderly, the most common urological and gynaecological procedures performed in old, or even very old patients are mainly endoscopic or perineal procedures: TURP or of bladder tumours, desobstruction of the urinary tract including placement or change of ureteral prosthesis, cure of phimosis, endoscopic uretrotomies, bladder neck incision, subalbugineous orchidectomy (pulpectomy), prostatic biopsies, treatment of urinary incontinence in women (transobturator or transvaginal tapes, various surgical cures of cystocele, rectocele or urogenital prolapse, LeFort colpocleisis, vaginal hysterectomies), and in men (artificial urinary sphincter placement), and peritoneal dialysis catheter placement in terminal renal failure patients.

For most of these procedures, the choice between general and regional (mainly spinal) anaesthesia must be discussed considering the specific medical condition of the patient and his/her wishes.

Infection of the urinary tract is always a threat, specifically in obstructive diseases and in patients with permanent bladder catheters.

Trans-urethral resection of the prostate conveys risks not only of specific 'TURP syndrome' but also of haemorrhage (a risk also associated to trans-urethral resection of bladder tumours and to supra or retro pubic adenomectomy). Very often in the elderly on anticoagulants or anti-platelet treatment a delicate balance is to be found between the importance of these treatments and the necessity to limit the haemorrhagic consequences of surgery.

Placement of peritoneal dialysis catheters often brings on the challenge of anaesthetizing very old, frail, patients with terminal renal failure.

10.2 **TURP surgery**

TURP is a very common surgical procedure, representing more than a third of all urological surgery. It is performed by introducing in the bladder a urethroscope and resecting prostatic tissue with an electrically powered metal loop which coagulates while resecting. The procedure usually lasts around one hour and is performed in the lithotomy position. Prostate is an organ rich in blood supply, and it usually harbours a significant amount of bacteria difficult to eradicate since the penetration of most antibiotics in this tissue is poor. TURP can be proposed to alleviate the obstruction created by a prostatic adenoma, but in the elderly the obstruction may also be due to advanced prostatic cancer.

The long-term mortality after TURP has been estimated around 15–20% in several studies. Nevertheless when compared with a cohort of matched non-operated individuals, the mortality risk was not increased by TURP (Cattolica, *J. Urol.*, 1997). Therefore, the outcome depends mainly on co-morbidities. Nevertheless, some complications may occur and steps should be taken to reduce their incidence and severity.

10.2.1 **Infection**

Bacteraemia are very frequent during urinary tract surgery, and it is mandatory not to operate on non-sterile urine. Nevertheless, when germs are present at the pre-operative urine analysis, the current tendency is to shorten (down to 12 hours) the duration of pre-operative antibiotic treatment in an asymptomatic patient devoid of pre-operative indwelling catheter provided the choice of the antibiotic is based on an antibiogram. Even if the urines are sterile, it is the rule to administer a single dose of prophylactic antibiotic intravenously on arrival in the operation room, dose which may be repeated every 2 hours while surgery is ongoing. The nature of the antibiotic depends on the ecology of the hospital, but second generation cephalosporins (i.e. cefamandole) are the most common choice.

In the presence of a chronic indwelling catheter, the risk of urine colonisation is very high, and it is difficult to get rid of the germs as long as the catheter is present. Before surgery, patients with chronic indwelling catheters should receive an antibiotic treatment adapted to the germs found in the urine, not so much to eradicate the infection but rather to render the blood "hostile" to those bacteria and therefore prevent bacteraemia and further infectious consequences.

10.2.2 **TURP syndrome**

The TURP syndrome is a clinical and biological entity due to excessive absorption of irrigation solution, usually glycine 1.5%. Irrigation solutions used intra-operatively are purposely moderately hypotonic to improve visualisation of the surgical site and must not have any electrical conductivity since the technique is based on electrocautery. As a consequence, when a significant amount enters the blood stream, fluid overload and hyponatraemia occur. The symptoms are those of hypervolaemia associated with water intoxication. As soon as the diagnosis is suspected, an urgent treatment should be initiated: interruption of surgery as early as possible (haemostasis!); replacement of glycine by saline in the irrigation solution; administration of diuretics to alleviate fluid overload (in serious cases, catecholamines may be required to sustain the heart). Plasma sodium concentration should be repeatedly checked; if it remains over 120 μmol L^{-1}, restricting water input and diuretics are usually enough. In case of deep hyponatraemia, that is when plasma sodium concentration less than 120 μmol L^{-1}, careful infusion of hypertonic saline may be required, keeping in mind that some authors consider that a too rapid correction may lead to neurological complications (central demyelinisation). Glycine by itself has toxic effects mainly on the heart and retina. Nevertheless, glycine toxicity is uncommon among TURP patients.

Specifically in elderly frail patients, TURP syndrome is dangerous and should be prevented. The French Health Authorities (1998) have noted the following guidelines for the prevention of TURP syndrome:

- Surgery should not last more than 60 minutes.
- Limit hydrostatic pressure in the bladder by allowing no more than 2 ft difference in height between the bladder and the irrigation pouch.

- Use double stream optic resectors to permit a continuous drainage of the bladder content.
- Limit the extent of the resection (the amount of reabsorbed fluid is proportional to the amount of resected tissue) (see Box 10.1).

Box 10.1 Prevention of TURP complications in the elderly

- Do not operate on non-sterile urines, use antibiotic prophylaxis.
- Limit the duration of resection to 60 minutes.
- The cut-off volume of the prostate for TURP is approximately 60–80 g. If higher, suprapubic adenomectomy should be performed.
- Limit hydrostatic pressure in the bladder.
- Control blood loss and transfuse if necessary.

10.2.3 **Bladder perforation and rupture**

Accidental perforation of the bladder during endoscopic urological surgery is rare but may happen either due to surgical instrumentation or due to over-distension of the bladder. Most of the time, the perforation is retroperitoneal. An early sign of this complication is the decreased return of the irrigation fluid from the bladder. Later, if under regional anaesthesia, the patient may experience abdominal distension and distress, hypotension and nausea. When the perforation is instrumental, the surgeon is usually aware of it. Immediate suprapubic bladder suture is advocated.

10.2.4 **Bleeding**

Trans-urethral resections of both prostates and bladder tumours often lead to significant haemorrhage. This risk is further increased by anticoagulant or anti-platelet treatments, very frequent in the elderly (see below). The exact amount of blood lost is difficult to estimate intra-operatively due to the constant irrigation, and blood replacement will be based on haemoglobin concentration or haematocrit measurement. In the elderly, a haemoglobin concentration under $10 \text{ g } 100 \text{ ml}^{-1}$ usually requires blood transfusion. At the end of the procedure, a significant hypovolaemia may exist, and the transition from the lithotomy to the supine position must be progressive, one leg at a time to avoid dangerous hypotension. In the post-operative period, irrigation is carried on with saline in order to avoid intravesical blood clots which may lead to re-operation for emptying the bladder and haemostasis. New surgical techniques (photoselective vaporisation of the prostate, green laser) may reduce this problem in the near future.

10.2.5 The elderly patient taking anti-platelet or anticoagulant drugs and presented for endoscopic urological surgery

Anti-platelet therapy has become a major treatment for both coronary artery disease and stroke. As a consequence, several millions of people are thus treated in Western Europe, the vast majority being elderly patients. Furthermore, smoking is an important contributive factor of both atherosclerosis and bladder tumours. Thus, having to anaesthetise an elderly patient on anti-platelet drugs for an endoscopic urological procedure is a frequent situation.

Interrupting such a treatment is associated with a real risk of severe coronary event, occurring with a mean delay of 11 days, time to recovery of platelet function. In the month which follows coronary stent implantation, temporary interruption in the patient taking one or both anti-platelet drugs translates to a risk of death through stent thrombosis of approximately 25%. To reduce this risk, it is necessary to wait at least 6 weeks after stent implantation to propose a temporary interruption at least partial of the treatment. The risk of stent thrombosis is even higher when coated stents have been used.

On the other hand, endoscopic urologic procedures are associated with significant bleeding which may threaten life. In the post-operative period, this bleeding may require surgical clot removal and haemostasis. Bleeding and its consequences are significantly increased in patients under anti-platelet treatment.

There are no completely satisfying solutions for this problem, even if new surgical approaches are promising. In all cases, adenosine diphosphate (ADP) receptor inhibitors (clopidogrel, ticlopidine) should be interrupted and replaced if mandatory by low-dose aspirin. Aspirin itself should be interrupted 4 or 5 days before surgery to associate some recovery of platelet function and some minimal protective anti-platelet residual effect. The interest of substitution (low-molecular-weight heparin [LMWH], short half-life non-steroidal anti-inflammatory drugs [NSAIDs] such as flurbiprofen) therapy is controversial since its efficiency is not proven and it may delay resuming the former treatment. The decision should always result from a discussion between the cardiologist (or neurologist), the anaesthetist and the surgeon and be recorded in the patient's file.

When the pre-operative evaluation leads to the discovery of a coronary stenosis requiring stent implantation, the discussion may arise to perform the endoscopic urological procedure under β-blockers and statins, delaying the stent implantation till after surgery.

As far as oral anticoagulants are concerned, they should always be interrupted before urological endoscopic surgery. A substitution by a more manageable drug depends on the indication for anticoagulation.

Patients with metallic mitral valves and at a lesser degree metallic aortic valves and patients suffering from atrial fibrillation usually receive a substitution treatment by heparin in the peri-operative period.

10.3 Endoscopic or perineal urological or gynaecological surgery in the elderly, which anaesthesia?

In most anaesthesia textbooks, the interest of spinal anaesthesia has been outlined in this situation: the act is technically simple, the lithotomy or gynaecologic position limits the haemodynamic consequences of the sympathetic blockade and the patient remaining conscious allows rapid diagnosis of complications such as ruptured bladder or TURP syndrome. In the treatment of urinary incontinence by sub-urethral tapes, some surgeons prefer the patient to remain conscious and be able to cough when asked to optimize the tension of the tape. Other surgeons stress that this adjustment on cough is useless, since patients are not expected to void in gynaecologic position. New anaesthetic agents and techniques have somehow tilted the balance back towards general anaesthesia, specifically in cases in which difficulties may arise with spinal. In patients on anticoagulants or anti-platelet therapy, even if spinal anaesthesia is not directly contraindicated in all cases, the risk of complications must be discussed and the reason spinal anaesthesia is chosen should be recorded in the patient's file. The risk of medullar haematoma is increased by the technical difficulties, and the technique should be abandoned if not successful at the first attempt. In patients with hypertension and/or cardiac failure, it is often easier to maintain haemodynamic stability with general anaesthesia. In rheumatic patients, the gynaecologic position sustained for more than 30 minutes may generate backache or pain in the lower limbs which may be attributed to spinal anaesthesia thus inducing complaints and litigation.

If general anaesthesia is chosen, a simple and efficient solution is to use a laryngeal mask with pressure support ventilation. Hypnosis can be maintained either with propofol target controlled infusion (TCI) (Schnider's model) or volatiles (preferably desflurane or sevoflurane), and analgesia is achieved with a rapid action opioid (alfentanil or remifentanil) in order to adjust the opioid to the respiratory rate (around 10–12 min^{-1}). Prostatic biopsies are usually performed under local anaesthesia, but if necessary some degree of conscious sedation may be used (propofol TCI, target around 1 μg ml^{-1}). Changes of ureteral prosthesis in women can also be performed under local anaesthesia, but a low target remifentanil TCI can significantly improve the acceptance of the technique.

Further reading

Burger W, Chemnitius JM, Kneissl GD and Rucker G. Low-dose aspirin for secondary cardiovascular prevention – cardiovascular risks after its perioperative withdrawal versus bleeding risks with its continuation – review and meta-analysis. *J Intern Med* 2005; **257**: 399–414.

Cattolica, EV, Sidney, and Sadler, MC. The safety of transurethral prostatectomy: a Cohort Study of Mortality in 9,416 men. *J. Urol.* 1997. **158** (1): 102–4

Grabe, M. Perioperative antibiotic prophylaxis in urology. *Curr Opin Urol* 2001; **11**: 81–85.

Hahn RG. Fluid absorption in endoscopic surgery. *Br J Anaesth* 2006; **96**: 8–20.

Seki N and Naito S. Instrumental treatments for benign prostatic obstruction. *Curr Opin Urol* 2007; **17**: 17–21.

Chapter 11

Post-operative care and analgesia

Key points

- Delayed recovery is mainly due to residual effects of anaesthetic agents/pre-medication.
- Emergence delirium may be dangerous and should be recognised and treated as an emergency.
- Spectacles and hearing aids should be given back as soon as possible on the recovery phase.
- Pain and its intensity may be difficult to recognize and quantify in the elderly, but there are no data to sustain the idea of a reduced perception of pain.
- Increased inter-individual variability requires titration to effect rather than a fixed dosage, and when the mental status of the patient allows it, patient controlled analgesia (PCA) is quite appropriate.

11.1 Post-operative care in the elderly

Intermediate recovery is a dangerous period when resuming of autonomy for vital functions of the patient allows close monitoring to shift towards less individualized care, but the patient cannot yet be safely left alone. Ideally, the mental status and awareness of the environment regain their pre-operative values, cardiovascular and respiratory function are stabilized, and pain and post-operative nausea and vomiting (PONV) are controlled. Unfortunately, this may take a long time, specifically in the elderly, and often inter-current obstacles need be got over.

11.2 Delayed recovery

Astonishingly enough, delayed recovery has not been extensively investigated, perhaps for lack of clear definition. In intubated patients, delayed recovery may be considered if removal of tracheal tube is impossible owing to altered consciousness (Glasgow score <9). In a case of delayed recovery, the first step is to protect the patient mainly from the respiratory consequences of this coma (aspiration of gastric content, obstructive apnoea). The airway must be protected and if necessary ventilation controlled to normal oxygen and $P_{ET}CO_2$ levels.

Delayed recovery may have two major causes: excessive residual sedation or neurological complication. Elderly patients are particularly exposed to both. Neurological complications leading to delayed recovery are mainly stroke (ischemic or haemorrhagic) and epilepsy. Strokes are very rare in the post-operative period outside of cardiac, intracranial or carotid surgeries. Convulsions may be triggered by metabolic disturbances (hypomagnesaemia, hypocalcaemia). Most of the time, delayed recovery is due to excessive sedation by residual action of sedative drugs used either intra-operatively or as a pre-medication. Thus, midazolam even at low doses or clonidine used as pre-medication may delay recovery in elderly patients. This increased risk of residual sedation reinforces the recommendation to favour short acting titrable anaesthetic agents in this population (Box 11.1).

Akinesia due to interruption of treatment in severe Parkinson's disease patients may mimic delayed recovery. For long surgery, it may be useful to consider dispersible enteric forms of LevoDopa immediately before surgery.

Box 11.1 Guidelines for aetiological diagnosis of delayed recovery

- Hypoxaemia? Check monitoring.
- Severe hypo- or hypercapnia?
- Chock? Profound anaemia?
- Residual action of hypnotic drugs? Of opioids? Residual muscle relaxation? Check anaesthesia sheet.
- Hypothermia?
- Chronic treatment by clonidine or lithium?
- Nature and dose of pre-medication?
- Neurological state: Glasgow score, focal neurologic signs? Pupil size and reactivity?
- Is the patient at risk for epilepsia?
- Metabolic disturbances (hypoglycaemia, severe acidosis, etc.)
- Central anticholinergic syndrome.

11.3 **Emergence delirium**

Emergence delirium in the post-anaesthetic care unit (PACU) remains poorly understood. It can become dangerous (self-inflicted injuries, haemorrhage, self-extubation and removal of catheters), requiring physical and chemical restraint. Age is a significant contributive factor, as well as linguistic problems, chronic alcoholism, previously altered mental status, depression or Parkinson's disease. If the lingering effect of anaesthetic agents rather leads to sedation, a poor recovery of consciousness associated with significant pain may trigger agitation. Patients on chronic benzodiazepine treatment are also more likely to develop emergence delirium even in the absence of proper withdrawal syndrome. Traditionally, anticholinergic agents have been accused to trigger agitation in the elderly. It remains a very minor causative factor in the PACU.

11.4 **Causative factors for PACU agitation**

The first step is to eliminate obvious causes.

11.4.1 **Post-operative urinary retention (POUR)**

Retention of urine is a common post-operative problem, and it may lead to agitation and confusion until relief is brought by bladder catheterisation. Age is an independent risk factor for POUR (the risk is doubled after 60 years), as well as amount of intra-operative fluids and bladder volume on entry in the PACU. Considering the alterations of urodynamics physiology with ageing, a single episode of POUR, if not rapidly treated, may increase the risk of further retentions. Patients arriving in the PACU with an intravesical volume of more than 270 ml represent half of the patients having received with more than 750 ml of intra-operative fluids. Of them, 30% will have a POUR in PACU. Other significant factors are sex (male, and the responsibility of undiagnosed prostatic adenoma is likely), large intra-operative opioid doses and central blockade including epidural analgesia.

11.4.2 **Pain**

Excruciating pain will generate agitation and must be treated as an emergency.

11.4.3 **Obstruction of a tracheal tube**

The other aetiologies must be checked out in the order of emergency.

Hypoxia is less frequent nowadays when supplemental oxygen is widely used and tissue oxygenation monitored through pulse oximetry.

Hypotension may reduce brain perfusion pressure, specifically in patients with history of stroke.

The metabolic disorders which may trigger agitation are mainly hypoglycaemia (diabetic patients, liver failure), hyponatraemia (TURP syndrome) and hypercalcaemia.

Sepsis. More than 20% of patients suffering from sepsis show agitation and confusion. Similarly, unexplained agitation after intra-abdominal surgery hints at surgical complications.

Residual paralysis. Even after a single intubating dose of non-depolarising muscle relaxant and in the absence of reversal, as much as 45% of patients admitted in PACU had a train of four (TOF) ratio inferior to 90% (Debaene, *Anesthesiology* 2003). Considering the fact that the clinical duration of action of most neuromuscular blocking agents (NMBA) is prolonged in the elderly, reversal should be the rule in this population as well as instrumental monitoring of muscle relaxation in all situations in which a muscle relaxant has been used.

Panic when awakening in a foreign environment may trigger or exacerbate agitation. It is worsened by the absence of spectacles and hearing aids, a poor pre-operative communication with the medical team, and pain.

11.5 **Treatment**

Once the above-mentioned aetiologies have been considered and treated, symptomatic treatment of persisting agitation is often necessary.

The patient should be, if possible, placed in a quiet environment, and the number of staff in direct relation with him/her should be reduced.

In a non-communicant elderly, reassuring words may not be sufficient.

Benzodiazepines are difficult to handle in the post-operative period, specifically in the elderly and if the patient has received opioids for pain, they may precipitate a dangerous respiratory depression. So, they should be ruled out unless a withdrawal syndrome is suspected. Neuroleptics and specifically haloperidol are the choice treatment even if their IV administration is not admitted in every country. The initial dosage is 5 mg injected slowly to be repeated every 15 minutes until the desired effect is achieved.

11.6 **Post-operative analgesia in the elderly**

The elderly patient does not require a complete change in the management of post-operative pain treatment but rather an adaptation of the usual practice to meet the specific requirements in this population.

11.6.1 **Perception and expression of pain in the elderly**

Pain and its intensity may be difficult to recognize and quantify in the elderly due to an atypical expression. Elderly patients usually ask for less analgesic drugs than their younger counterparts, but this does not necessarily mean a less intense perception of pain. Pharmacology of analgesic drugs in this population will lead to a reduction in doses and their frequency. Cultural and sociological background may induce a more restrained expression of discomfort, and even in the absence of real confusion, visual and/or hearing impairment may cut the elderly off from the environment and reduce communication.

11.6.2 **Measuring pain in the elderly**

The use of very common assessment tools (VAS for example) may be rendered difficult in visually impaired or confused patients. To improve communication, spectacles and hearing aids should be given back to the elderly patient as soon as possible on the recovery phase. In children, comportment scales are used to bypass the communication problem. These scales have not so far been formalized in the elderly. Their applicability is reduced by the fact that the evaluation of pain by nurses and doctors may be very different from what the patient perceives, and more so in the elderly. Nevertheless, physiological parameters (blood pressure, heart rate, respiratory rate) and facial expression may help (Box 11.2).

11.6.3 **Pharmacology of analgesic drugs in the elderly**

Practitioners are often reticent to prescribe potent analgesics in the elderly under the false assumption that the treatment might be more dangerous than pain itself. A key feature of ageing is the enhancement of inter-individual variability. Therefore a titration to effect will always be better than a fixed dosage, and when the mental status of the patient allows it, PCA is quite appropriate.

11.6.3.1 *Opioids*

The concentration–effect relationship of all opioids is modified in the elderly, and, as a consequence, the efficient opioid concentrations are reduced approximately by half in this population. Therefore, even in the absence of pharmacokinetic changes, the bolus doses of morphine should be divided by two in the elderly. Renal failure is associated with accumulation of the glucuronide active metabolites. Urinary retention after morphine administration is more frequent in the elderly, specifically in male patients and should be called to mind when agitation increases despite adequate pain relief.

> **Box 11.2 Pain evaluation by the nursing team in non-communicant patients**
>
> **Level 1:** Calm, relaxed facial features, may be sleeping, normal respiratory rate, normal heart rate, no hypertension
> **Level 2:** Anxious, tense, tachypnoeic, tachycardiac
> **Level 3:** Agitated or prostrated, moaning either spontaneously or when touched, tachycardiac, hypertensive, sweating

11.6.3.2 NSAIDs

Non-steroidal anti-inflammatory drugs (NSAIDs) are very efficient painkillers, including in the elderly. Unfortunately their use is associated with a number of unwanted side effects among which the most troublesome in aged patients is the reduction in glomerular filtration rate which may precipitate acute renal failure. Therefore, the dose should be reduced and their use should be limited in time in this population. Cox2-inhibitors, the clinical use of which has been restrained by its cardiovascular impact, have the same renal action as other NSAIDs.

11.6.3.3 Acetaminophen (paracetamol), nefopam

Acetaminophen can be readily used in elderly patients, alone or as part of a multi-modal analgesic protocol. The dosage is the same as in younger patients, 1 g every 6 hours. Its onset is slow, and the first dose should be given intra-operatively to be effective at recovery.

Nefopam may also be included in a multi-modal analgesic protocol. Its use has no specificity in the elderly.

11.6.3.4 Tramadol

Tramadol may also be very useful in the elderly. Its elimination is reduced in elderly patients as a consequence of impaired renal function. In addition, its active metabolite may accumulate. As a consequence, the interval of time between two doses should be doubled.

11.6.4 Regional analgesia

Regional analgesia may be very profitable in elderly patients. It provides an excellent pain relief without interfering with consciousness. Peripheral blockade, when applicable, is particularly well suited to this population. It can induce a very long post-operative analgesia and sometimes even create concerns for a persistent neurological deficit so much so that pre-existing neuropathies have not always been documented pre-operatively (trauma patients). Central blockade is more questionable. It may impair early perambulation and be associated with hypotension and urinary retention.

11.6.5 Consequences of pain and its treatment on post-operative course

Pain per se may have deleterious effects. It is a factor of confusion (see above), and of cardiac and respiratory complications. Conversely, an efficient analgesia is beneficial in frail patients as well as in others. In orthopaedic surgery, it allows a more effective physiotherapy and an earlier perambulation.

The treatment of pain should be integrated into a wider rehabilitation program to help the elderly resume his/her activities as soon as possible.

Further reading

Aubrun F. Management of postoperative analgesia in elderly patients. *Reg Anesth Pain Med* 2005; **30**: 363–379.

Debaene B, Plaud B, Dilly MP and Donati F. Residual paralysis in the PACU after a single intubating dose of nondepolarizing muscle relaxant with an intermediate duration of action. *Anesthesiology* 2003; **98**: 1042–1048.

Fong HK, Sands LP and Leung JM. The role of postoperative analgesia in delirium and cognitive decline in elderly patients: A systematic review. *Anesth Analg* 2006; **102**: 1255–1266.

Fredman B, Lahav M, Zohar E, Golod M, Paruta I and Jedeikin R. The effect of midazolam premedication on mental and psychomotor recovery in geriatric patients undergoing brief surgical procedures. *Anesth Analg* 1999; **89**: 1382–1387.

Keita H, Diouf E, Tubach F, Brouwer T, *et al*. Predictive factors of early postoperative urinary retention in the postanesthesia care unit. *Anesth Anag* 2005; **101**: 592–596.

Chapter 12

Intensive care and the elderly

Key points

- The elderly are more likely to need intensive care than younger patients.
- Survival is a poor indicator of outcome.
- Pre-existing organ reserve determines outcome.
- End-of-life decisions have to be made prior to admission.
- Prolongation of dying is an ever-present risk.
- Nearly 50% of all UK intensive care patients are over 65.
- Advanced directives often include some restriction in intensive care management.
- Medical admissions are higher risk than surgical admissions.

12.1 Background

Intensive care across the world is expensive – it currently costs 1% of the gross domestic product (GDP) of the USA. The utilisation of intensive care by the elderly has increased in line with the changes in demography. More than 27% of all UK admissions are for patients over 75 years of age. This has an influence on expected outcome because of the progressive changes in physiological performance of organ systems and total body homeostasis (see Chapter 2). For example, in patients over the age of 85, less than 10% can reach an anaerobic threshold of >11 ml s kg^{-1} min^{-1}. This is the value at which patients enter the 'high risk' stratification for major abdominal surgery with a predicted mortality of >18%.

Behavioural adaptation to the progressive decline in physiological reserve is normal for the elderly and they begin to restrict what they do to the limits of their functional capability. This is often implicit and the patients do not recognize that they have changed their pattern of life. For example, they go shopping only with their children (exercise or cognitive function), take relatives or close friends to all social events including attending out-patient departments (cognitive function) or fluid restrict because of bladder or mobility problems. Simple enquiry from relatives may be more productive than seeking the answers directly from the patient.

Discrimination is an integral part of clinical practice and forms the basis of allocating resources to those who are likely to gain the most benefit from them. This is clearly a difficult area because the basis of this discrimination can be very variable. One of the many possible criteria used to make these choices is age. The rational approach would be one that tried to identify and quantify the outcome of applying a finite resource to a given problem. How long should we provide ventilatory support for this patient with severe pneumonia? Will they survive and get back to work?

When countries spend much more on the health care of the elderly (Finland spends 5.5% more on people over 65 years of age than on those under 65) a case for increased spending on prevention in the young rather than intensive care for the elderly could be made.

12.2 Outcome

Outcome from admission to an intensive care unit is going to be determined by these influences regardless of the cause. There are simple outcome measures that are of limited value. These include mortality. Survival is a binary code and it is worth remembering that having a good death may be the best option for the patients and their family.

The number of patients over 70 years who survive for more than 3 months after an ICU admission is only 50% (Table 12.1). This doubling in mortality from acute illness to discharge reflects both the frailty of the patients and their limited reserve to recover from the major demands that illness places on their metabolism.

Table 12.1 Survival data on patients leaving ITU and at 3 months – impact of age		
Age	Discharge from ITU (%)	3-month survival (%)
75–79	68	54
80–84	75	56
>85	69	51

Survival has also to be weighed against the normal pattern of life expectancy and the survival effect. Life expectancy is almost static at about a 50% – 5 years survival from the age of 65 onwards. A 90-year-old still has a life expectancy of 5 years! This is because the frail and infirm have already died and only the tough (and lucky) have survived.

Better measures of outcome relate to the function of the patient in terms of their pre-admission status. This may be assessed across a large number of domains, but they usually include those relating to cognitive or neurophysiological status, activities of daily living or handicap. In general, patients who survive for more than 3 months also have a reasonable functional outcome, although this may simply be another way of defining the same thing; patients who can recover well also survive. There are 'geriatric' scoring systems that show that over 90% of survivors get back to their social environment, but only about two-thirds regain their activities of daily living. This may be due to the short-time frame of the surveys because many elderly take more than 6 months to recover from intermediate level surgery. Getting over major surgery or overwhelming infection is likely to take longer still.

Serious pre-existing illnesses such as congestive cardiac failure, dementia, malnutrition or diabetes all limit functional recovery.

Quality of life is a very personal but often assessed as an outcome measure. When elderly patients were reviewed after ICU admission, many thought they had a good quality of life despite reduced function. The alternatives may have been seen to be worse but these findings do indicate that subjective assessments by the care team of what the quality of life may be should not be used to decide on treatment plans.

12.3 Technology

Advances in organ support systems over the last few decades have meant that more patients, the elderly included, will survive for longer than they would have done without this support. This process may extend dying rather than allowing recovery and can be inappropriate in some patients. It is for these reasons among others that clinical review of all patients is recommended before admission to intensive care units. The key decisions to be made are related to the likely benefit to the patient of such an admission, and their own wishes (even if admission were to be of value). This may be difficult if there is missing information on the presenting clinical condition or other underlying disease states, such as malignancy, that may influence likely prognosis.

Where identified these may indicate limiting intensive care either by time or by intervention. Some patients expressly reject ventilation as being a step too far, others wish for a 'Do Not Attempt to Resuscitate' (DNAR) to be enacted with immediate effect. It is more unusual in the elderly for the family to wish to 'have everything done'.

Patients who present severely ill from a medical cause have a different prognosis to those admitted with either a surgical or traumatic cause. The latter are likely to have a condition that is improved by the surgery, valve replacement surgery for example, or a fractured pelvis after fixation. Acute exacerbations of chronic illnesses such as severe pulmonary oedema on a background of ischaemic heart disease will have a limited chance of recovery of function. As more of acute care is interventional rather than surgical so has the proportion of medical admissions to ICU increased and may be as high as 80% in unselected admissions units.

One area of intensive care that has a positive benefit to elderly surgical patients is in the pre-operative aggressive management to optimize their oxygen delivery prior to surgery. This 'goal-directed' care improves clinical outcome and survival at all ages. At present it is routinely used in only a few units in the UK but is likely to become more widespread as pressure on ICU and surgical beds continues to mount.

12.4 **Futility**

As the patient's response to treatment in progress or being planned is reviewed, it is important to assess whether there has been or is likely to be any benefit from the treatment. On one level this is about causing minimum harm to the patient and on the other about not prolonging the act of dying. This is clearly good medical practice and should be common across all areas of clinical practice. However, this is a frequent event within intensive care units and most units have clear protocols for the withdrawal of treatment based on the latest General Medical Council UK (GMC) guidance.

Accepting that further clinical care is futile is very difficult for many practitioners, and often for the close family of the patient. Actively moving to provide palliative care for these patients is one avenue, whereas the dignified withdrawal of active measures may be another.

Convincing the current elderly cohort of patients that medicine does not provide immortality is usually straightforward but the over-optimistic portrayal of recovery from near death on TV programmes is confusing for their relatives and younger family members. Creating enough time to educate them into understanding reality may be hard. On occasion this makes it difficult to move from treatment to palliation. The timing of implementation of these decisions will depend on the acceptance by the patient and their family that there is no further benefit to be gained and that further systems support will only prolong the process of dying. This may take no time at all or several days. During the latter process, the care team will also need emotional support to continue what they may believe is unnecessary interventional management.

One of the most extreme and pressing situations for the assessment of futility is when a cardiac arrest occurs in hospital. This frequently involves elderly patients who have significant pre-existing medical problems. The success of resuscitation leading to discharge from hospital is very low. Approximately 15% of all patients will survive, but this falls with increasing age. No survivors are likely after the age of 70, although they may be resuscitated enough to be admitted to ICU. Of those who are admitted, 50% have significant neurological damage and the others develop depression or other stress-related disorders.

In the face of these dreadful outcomes, many elderly patients choose to enact DNAR in the event of a cardiac arrest. These wishes may be formally communicated by the patient or more informally through their relatives. If the ward staff are not aware of these DNAR records, resuscitation will be attempted.

12.5 **Complications**

There are many complications due to the complex nature of the multi-organ support that may be necessary for the elderly patient, but these are usually short lived and related to either practical interventions or drug therapy. Some however are responsible for prolonged disability and loss of independence. These include post-operative cognitive dysfunction and sleep disorders (see Chapter 5). They may be physical, psychological and social problems. Unlike younger patients, once these complications arise they may prove insurmountable.

Weight loss and muscle loss are common after prolonged immobilization. Partly due to the catabolism and poor nutrition, this limits the patient's ability to mobilize and, especially in the elderly, increases the convalescence time. Further muscular dysfunction affects the diaphragm and intercostal muscles. This results in breathlessness on exertion as well as a predisposition to respiratory complications due to inefficient coughing and sputum clearance. Sensory and motor neuropathies may occur, as can alterations in the special senses of sight, smell and hearing. If the airway has been instrumented – tracheostomy/endotracheal tube – for a length of time, then tracheal stenosis, vocal cord damage or stridor may occur.

Patients often have difficulty in relating back into their social grouping, whether family or care home. This may be as a result of their experiences during admission or subtle cognitive changes as a result of the illness and therapies needed for recovery.

12.6 **Advanced directives/capacity**

Increasing numbers of elderly patients have chosen what level of medical care they wish to receive if they become incapacitated. In the UK, this has recently been updated to rationalize the 'power of attorney' legally granted (often to relatives) to carers to enable decisions of medical treatment as well as financial and other matters to be made in the best interests of the patient. Historically many of these powers were abused, although this was usually in the financial arena for self-gain (see Chapter 14).

What is important is to adopt the position that all elderly patients will have an advanced directive until proven otherwise. Finding the details may be difficult, as they may have spoken only to close relatives rather than committing their wishes to paper. Acting in the best interests of the patient until these can be identified is reasonable, but once known they must be followed to avoid the risk of litigation. The most common stipulation is in the case of needing resuscitation, but may include the prohibition of naso-gastric tubes, catheterisation or even palliative operations.

12.7 **Summary**

The elderly are the most expensive users of intensive care facilities, and many gain tremendous benefit from their admission. This is more likely if their reason for admission is surgical or traumatic than if an underlying medical cause exists. Common sense has to balance the ability to do something with the question of appropriateness.

Further reading

Hutton P, Cooper GM, James III FM and Butterworth IV JF Eds (2002). *Fundamental Principles and Practice of Anaesthesia.* Martin Dunitz Ltd, UK IABN 1-899066-57-8. Chapter 17.

Chapter 13

Cognitive dysfunction and sleep disorders

113

> ## Key points
>
> - Of all patients over the age of 65 undergoing major surgery, 25% will have a degree of cognitive impairment.
> - Eleven per cent will have permanent changes.
> - Up to 73% of elderly surgical patients will have an episode of delirium.
> - Assessment of mental function is a core skill for all doctors.
> - Knowledge of the causes and treatment of delirium are necessary.
> - Evidence for the superiority of any one anaesthetic technique is lacking.
> - Elderly patients who complain of cognitive decline after surgery should be taken seriously.
> - Cognitive impairment is associated with poor peri-operative pain control.

13.1 Size of the problem

The most devastating complication following surgery is that due to changes in cognition. The incidence of post-operative cognitive dysfunction (POCD), although possible at any age, is greatest in the elderly. The elderly may suffer an acute episode such as delirium or a more chronic and slightly later onset of cognitive dysfunction. Both conditions are probably indications of loss of reserve of basic neuronal pathways such as the cholinergic or adrenergic systems (Table 13.1).

The identification of the more delayed form of POCD may be made once the patient returns home and may be missed by all but the close relatives of the patient. The incidence does not appear to

Table 13.1 Characteristics of delirium versus dementia		
Characteristic	**Delirium**	**Dementia**
Consciousness	Clouded Decreased or hyperalert	Usually alert
Orientation	Disorganized	Disoriented
Course	Fluctuating	Steady slow decline
Onset	Acute or subacute	Chronic
Attention	Impaired	Usually normal
Psychomotor	Agitated or lethargic	Usually normal
Hallucinations	Perceptual disturbances May have hallucinations	Usually not present
Sleep–awake cycle	Abnormal	Usually normal
Speech	Slow, incoherent	Usually normal, anomic difficulty finding words

Reproduced with permission from Flaherty JH (2006) Delirium. In: *Principles of Geriatric Medicine*, 4th edn, pp. 1047–1060. Sussex, England: John Wiley & Sons.

have changed over the last half century, at about 25% of all major surgical patients over the age of 65. This is despite all the changes in understanding, monitoring and newer anaesthetic agents with more benign pharmacodynamics.

13.2 **Delirium**

This is a medical emergency. It can occur within hours of surgery and often lasts up to 7 days. There are two sub-types of delirium: agitated and quiet. The former is much more likely to be diagnosed than the withdrawn quiet patient who appears simply compliant with instructions. The incidence of delirium in all hospital inpatients over the age of 65 averages about 35% and increases with advancing age, but depending on the type of surgery may rise to more than 70%.

There is a classification of delirium in the *Diagnostic and Statsitical Manual of Mental Disorders* (4th Ed, or DSM IV) which includes three forms:

1. Intoxication/withdrawal state

2. Multiple aetiology

3. General medical condition

It is the last one that is considered the most common form in hospitalized patients (Box 13.1).

Risk factors for developing delirium include advancing age, frailty, cognitive impairment or a previous episode of delirium. The last two can be confirmed by questioning the family when they may identify other episodes related to infections of minor trauma.

> ### Box 13.1 Criteria for medical causes of delirium (DSM IV) (APA, 1994)
>
> - Disturbance of consciousness (reduced clarity of awareness of the environment) with reduced ability to focus, sustain or shift attention.
> - A change in cognition (such as memory deficit, disorientation, language disturbance of perceptual disturbance) not better explained by a pre-existing or evolving dementia.
> - The disturbance develops over a short period of time (usually hours to days) and tends to fluctuate over the course of the day.
> - There is often evidence from the history, physical examination or laboratory findings that the disturbance is due to one or more medications or general medical conditions.

> ### Box 13.2 Precipitating factors for delirium
>
> - Hypoxia
> - Anticholinergic medication
> - Infective processes
> - Biochemical abnormalities
>   - Glucose/sodium/calcium
> - Centrally acting drugs
>   - Opiates
>   - Sedatives

The presenting symptoms are of acute and fluctuating changes in cognition and attention. The cognitive changes include disordered thinking, memory and perception while there changes in attention seen by reduced alertness, perception and directiveness. There is usually an alteration in their sleep/wake balance and patients become sleepy through the day and agitated during the nights. The agitation and disorientation suffered by these patients may lead to significant clinical problems, for example drains and intravenous lines can be pulled out or they may try to escape their frightening environment despite orthopaedic surgery requiring non-weight bearing. They are more likely to fall and further injure themselves.

The underlying cause is believed to involve the cholinergic pathways within the brain, although lymphokines have also been implicated and these will rise in infection, malignancy or following trauma. Precipitating factors have been identified, and suggested plans for identifying and managing delirium have been suggested (Boxes 13.2 and 13.3).

Box 13.3 Rockwood's 5-point plan for the management of delirium (Lindesay, 2002)

- Identify risk factors
  - Elderly, frail, very ill, prior history of dementia
- Treat reversible factors
  - Medication, infections, heart failure
- Keep control of the behaviours
  - Family vigils
- Anticipate problems
  - Full bladder/constipation, fall risks
- Prepare for rehabilitation

Box 13.4 Drug therapy for delirium

- Haloperidol
  - Oral (slow onset)/IM (fast onset)
    - Not for withdrawal patients
- Others – seek advice before using them
  - Atypical neuroleptics
    - Risperidone/olanzapine/quetiapine
  - Benzodiazepines
    - Lorazepam
  - Antidepressants
    - Trazadone

If patients have been identified as at increased risk for developing delirium, such as a previous episode or mild dementia, it may be worth involving the family to provide a 24- hour 'vigil' to maintain a personal orientation for the patient. Strict light/dark cycle (unlike most continuously well-lit wards) is maintained and cue to time and place, such as large obvious clocks and calendars, are provided.

Treatment of delirium lies in trying to identify the likely precipitating cause and drug therapy. Physical restraint is more likely to increase the level of harm and should never be disproportionate for safety. For example, it may be reasonable to temporarily restrain an arm to insert an IV cannula for drug administration but not to tether their arms to the cot sides.

The mainstay of drug therapy is haloperidol, IM or orally. As with all drugs in the elderly, the initial dose should be calculated in relation to their weight/age/sex and the severity of the delirium. Once a therapeutic response is achieved, the loading process should be stopped. Use of 'prn' doses should be reviewed as there may be a need to prescribe a regular, timed dose. The withdrawal of haloperidol should be gradual in case the underlying delirium is not resolved (Box 13.4).

Box 13.3 is reproduced with permission from Lindesay, J., Rockwood, K., and Macdonald, A. (2002). *Delirium in Old Age*. Oxford University Press, Newyork.

If haloperidol does not work, then expert advice from the psycho-geriatric service is necessary.

The outcome following an episode of delirium has serious implications for the patient. They have a much higher rate in the presentation of dementia than the normally ageing population (18% versus 5%) probably because it may be indicating a critically low functional reserve of cognitive function.

13.3 Post-operative cognitive dysfunction (POCD)

This is a condition that has been poorly defined yet recognized for more than 100 years as being a particular problem in anaesthetised elderly patients (Box 13.5). The concerns raised in the UK in the 1950s were of such magnitude that they effectively denied elderly patients any major surgery for decades. The evidence to date confirms that approximately 25% of all elderly having major surgery will have an identifiable fall in cognition. About half of these patients will have a permanent dysfunction. The risk increases with age, and indeed it is the main predictive factor.

The most common sign noticed by relatives is social disinhibition. The patient behaves in a mild but often embarrassingly different way than their usual form of behaviour. This may be as subtle as becoming irritated if kept waiting, or making personal remarks about strangers within their hearing. This may last for a week to several months. More pronounced changes such as loss of executive reasoning will leave them more dependent for support with simple tasks of daily living such as shopping.

Part of the problem with POCD and its incidence is related to the methods of testing for it. For a method of testing to be useful, it has to be given before and on several occasions after surgery. It should be reliable and consistent over all of these testing episodes with no learning effect from repeated testing. A large enough non-operative matched cohort should also be tested to identify the changes in a normal population over the same time epoch. This has led to many forms of testing and often heated discussions as to which is most appropriate (Figure 13.1).

Box 13.5 Features of POCD

- Cognitive changes that affect
  - Memory
  - Planning
  - Organization
  - Attention
  - Speed of information processing
  - Personality
    - Disinhibition

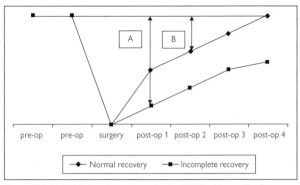

Figure 13.1 Typical design of a study examination POCD with a profile of normal recovery (diamonds) and incomplete recovery (squares) across multiple post-operative time points. Comparison A – change from baseline to post-op time point (incomplete recovery patient). Comparison B – change from baseline to post-op time point 2 (normal recovery patient).

The causes of POCD have been investigated over the years but no single cause is likely to explain the range and extent of the problem. The underlying biological basis is believed to be a cholinergic failure within the CNS (central nervous system) as the constellation of symptoms is very similar to Alzheimer's form of dementia. Hypoxia, hypotension, general anaesthesia are just a few of the causes that have been proposed but very large studies have failed to demonstrate that any of them is primarily to blame. Even the debate as to whether regional anaesthesia confers a greater safety margin than general anaesthesia is still unproven (Box 13.6).

One possible developing explanation may be the interaction that occurs after microglial and astrocyte activation that follows neuronal injury and the predisposition that astrocyte activation has for damage by a subsequent oxidative stress. This activated state can last for several months if not years. Many volatile and intravenous anaesthetic agents have actions on neuronal receptors, ranging from NMDA to cholinergic and adrenergic receptors. Some of these actions are protective and others depending on the concentration and the presence of mild hypoxia are damaging.

Assessment of the elderly patient's mental state is essential, not just to validate their consent to procedures, but also to check for any decrement following surgery. The simplest test is the abbreviated mental test (AMT) (Box 13.7) although the mini-mental state evaluation (MMSE) is more useful but takes up to 15 minutes to administer (Table 4.1).

This testing should be part of the core competencies of all doctors.

Figure 13.1 is reproduced from Lewis, M., Maruff, P., and Silbert, B. (2004). Statistical and conceptual issues in defining post-operative cognitive dysfunction. Neuroscience Biobehavioural Reviews **28**:433–40 with permission from Elsevier.

Box 13.6 Possible causes of POCD

- Hypoxia
- Hypotension
- General anaesthesia
- Stress responses
  - Central catecholamine changes
  - Steroid effects
- Central cholinergic (nicotinic) changes
- Age

Box 13.7 Abbreviated mental test (Hodkinson, 1972)

Age
Time (to the nearest hour)
Address – to recall at the end of the test:
42 West Street (ask patient to repeat the address to ensure it has been heard correctly)
Year
Name of hospital
Recognition of two persons (e.g. doctor, nurse)
Date of birth
Year of start of the First World War
Name of monarch
Count downwards from 20 to 1
Scores should be 9 or above

Treatment of POCD is difficult because it is uncertain as to what is the primary cause. Avoiding precipitating drugs such as the anticholinergic agents is imperative and close control of temperature, pain control and fluid balance is important. These are all known to increase the incidence of POCD. Cholinergic agonists have not been shown to have any benefit.

13.4 Sleep disorders

Disordered sleep is one of the almost inevitable consequences of getting older and there are several conditions that are prevalent in this age group. Even patients in their late nineties will have much the same duration of sleep in a 24-hour-period as their younger colleagues although the content and timing will have changed. The amount of deep slow wave sleep (SWS) (Stage 3–4) falls, but this may be due to the recording amplitude changes due to cell loss rather than actual changes in the pattern of sleep. The amount of rapid eye movement

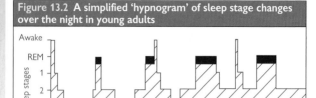

Figure 13.2 A simplified 'hypnogram' of sleep stage changes over the night in young adults

(REM) sleep, at about 20%, is also preserved. There are however changes in the amplitude of the circadian and ultradian rhythms with ageing.

The two main forms of sleep – slow wave and REM – have markedly different underlying physiological processes. SWS is an essentially stable state with brainstem control of all basic physiological processes such as breathing driven by arterial carbon dioxide concentrations. There are four 'stages' of increasing depth and during the latter two (SWS stage 3 + 4) many of the restorative cellular processes are believed to occur. Certainly these stages are when the anabolic hormones are largely released. REM sleep is an active state not dissimilar to being awake. Physiological processes react to mentation with the exception that most humans hyperpolarize their spinal motor tracts to cause paralysis during REM. This can fail and lead to sleep behavioural activity or not respond to wakening and thus lead to sleep paralysis. Whatever the dream, mentation includes physiology matches, dreams of running cause tachypnoea, tachycardia and hypertension; whereas swimming underwater leads to central apnoea. During both sleep patterns there is a progressive loss of motor power and this affects the upper airway as well (Figure 13.2) (see above).

13.5 Circadian changes

The normal sleep pattern of humans is regulated within the hippocampus and reinforced by light and dark cycling. For most people this is based on a 24-hour cycle. Within this pattern, there is further cyclical influence – the ultradian rhythm – which has a time base of about 60–90 minutes. This modulates the likelihood of being sleepy of awake within the slower sleep/wake cycling. As ageing occurs, these ultradian influences lead to larger oscillations within the circadian cycle and it becomes more common to feel sleepy during the day and wake through the night. By the age of 70, most people need an afternoon nap and wake at least once through the night.

The transition to very light sleep through the night means that somatic influences may allow the patient to break through into wakefulness. This is commonly seen where there is joint pain from arthritis for example. It may also make going to sleep more difficult. The normal timing of the sleep/wake cycle has been determined by the middle aged as going to sleep around midnight and waking at about 7:30 a.m. This is not true in either younger or older people. Teenagers do not start to feel sleepy until 2 a.m. in the morning and do not wake spontaneously until nearly noon. The elderly have moved forward and start to sleep at 10:00 and are wake at about 5–6 in the morning. This has an influence on when wards should dim the lights when older patients are admitted.

13.6 Anaesthetic/surgical influences on sleep

Sleep disturbance is universal on admission to hospital with the first night being at a much lighter plane of sleep than normal. There is complete suppression of both SWS and REM sleep. This also occurs on the first post-operative night, possibly exacerbated by opiates. There is marked rebound of SWS on the second and third nights with REM rebound occurring on later nights. The dramatic physiological surges related to REM sleep are believed to account for some of the late but severe complications such as myocardial ischaemia or stroke.

13.7 Episodic airway obstruction during sleep

One common problem in the elderly is that of repetitive airway obstruction during sleep. As ageing occurs the upper airway becomes increasing lax and the negative pressures necessary to initiate airflow during resting ventilation become enough to narrow the airway. If there is a marked constriction, snoring starts, and this affects almost 70% of all patients over 65 years. Further narrowing leads to louder snoring until ultimately the airway can be sucked shut. This leads to silence, but also increases efforts to breathe. The longer this continues, the lower the arterial oxygen tension will fall. Recovery is automatic and is due to brainstem arousal reactivating the pharyngeal constrictor muscles among others. This pattern is seen in obstructive sleep apnoea and in younger patients leads to hypersomnolence and an increased risk of right heart failure, stroke and cognitive dysfunction.

Box 13.8 **Examples of age-related sleep disorders**

- Insomnia
- Obstructive sleep apnoea
- Periodic limb movement disorder
- Restless legs syndrome
- Sleep phase advancement
- Hypersomnia – primary

This process does appear to be more benign in the elderly, and there is an increase in the number of episodes of obstruction with advancing age. However, they are rarely as sleepy as younger sufferers. It would still seem prudent to protect their airways as though they did have obstructive sleep apnoea. The falls in oxygen tension are very marked in these patients because of their reduced functional volumes and this does have an influence on wound healing (Box 13.8).

There are two other common conditions that become more prevalent with ageing: periodic limb movement (PLM) disorder and restless legs syndrome.

PLM may be present for many years but if it is first seen in later life it is frequently one of the very early signs of Parkinson's disease and referral to a neurologist for investigation is warranted. Drug therapy is usually very effective but is usually then a life-time treatment.

Restless legs syndrome may start at any age but is more common in the elderly. They describe a sensation of itching or burning under the skin on their legs that is improved by moving. It can be associated with a low serum iron and should be checked by assaying for serum ferritin levels before initiating treatment which may be with either ropinirole or pramipexole.

13.8 **Summary**

Disorders affecting cognition and sleep are common in the elderly. Some may have devastating consequences for the patient and their family yet we still know little about their causes and therefore opportunities to treat them.

Sleep disorders are also common and may have a different outcome in the elderly to younger patients.

Further reading

American Psychiatric Association. (1994) *The Diagnostic Statistical of Mental Disorders* 4th edn (DSM IV). The American Psychiatric Association, Washington DC.

Hodkinson HM. Evolution of a mental test score for assessment of mental impairment in the elderly. Age and Ageing. 1972; **1**: 233–8. Oxford University Press.

Kryger MH, Roth T and Dement W. (2005). *Principles and Practice of Sleep Medicine*, 4th edition (Principles & Practice of Sleep Medicine) ISBN 9780721607979, W.B. Saunders Co., UK.

Lindesay J, Rockwood K, and Macdonald A. (2002). *Delirium in Old Age*. Oxford University Press, New York.

Moller JT, Cluitmans P, Rasmussen LS, *et al.* ISPOCD investigators. Long-term postoperative cognitive dysfunction in the elderly: ISPOCD1 study. *Lancet* 1998; **351**: 857–861.

Rasmussen LS, Johnson T, Kuipers HM, et al. ISPOCD2 (International Study of Postoperative Cognitive Dysfunction) Investigators. Does anaesthesia cause postoperative cognitive dysfunction? A randomized study of regional versus general anaesthesia in 438 elderly patients. *Acta Anaesthesiol Scand* 2003 Mar; **47**(3): 260–266. PMID: 12648190.

Taylor M and Grant F. Cognitive dysfunctionin the elderly. Why assessment is of practical consequence to anaesthetists. *Curr Anaesth Crit Care* 2002; **13**: 221–227.

Chapter 14

Ethics and the law involving the elderly

> **Key points**
> - Ethics provide a system to judge whether care is for the individual's or society's benefit.
> - Ultimately ethical frameworks are the responsibility of society.
> - Duty of care follows from accepted ethical practice.
> - Consent is a process not a piece of paper.
> - Capacity may vary in time and degree.
> - Ethics demand that only an experienced doctor can take informed consent.
> - No-one else (except for children under 16) but the patient can give consent.
> - Information should be clearly provided and repeated often.
> - The elderly are often deaf, blind or both.

14.1 Ethics

The provision of health care throughout history has evolved by balancing the abilities of medical personnel (and their drugs/equipment etc.) with a society's willingness to tolerate their (the doctors) control over such fundamental issues as life or death. When the costs of providing such care are vast and the resources of the state limited, some degree of rationing has to take place. For this to be fair and just, decisions have to be made about who gets what. The elderly have a place in the society that also changes over time and place. In many parts of the world, they are venerated and respected whereas in others they are a burden.

Providing an equitable distribution of resources then has to be made somehow. It is in this arena that the use of ethics has such a pivotal role. Ethics are philosophical studies of the moral value of actions that is based on clear rules and principles. This philosophical debate has been adapted for use in clinical areas as 'codes of practice'. There are many sets of rules or theories in use, but the two common ones are 'Consequentialist or Utilitarianism' and 'Deontological'. These describe different process and intrinsically they are impractical ways of making daily decisions although they are usually both incorporated into our decision making.

In the Consequentialist approach, decisions are made simply on the balance of the risk of doing good rather than harm for each action. This ultimately leads to the possibility of doing the best for society rather than an individual. The Deontological process involves assessing the action itself against the individual rights, duties and need for justice. The consequences of the action are not considered.

Practically, ethics have been described as an 'analytical activity in which the concepts, assumption, beliefs, attitudes, emotions, reasons and arguments underlying medico-moral decision-making are examined critically'. It is a process that is usually described as being based on four principles:

1. Autonomy
2. Non-maleficence
3. Beneficence
4. Justice

Autonomy represents the individual's right to self-determination in all aspects of their life even if we do not agree with or share their beliefs. This is the cornerstone of consent – the giving and withholding according to the individuals choice. The principle that our actions should not be gratuitously harmful is enshrined in the second and implies that there has to be a balance between 'necessary harm' (such as surgery) for greater benefits. Beneficence is the act of doing good or behaving correctly in all dealings with patients, their families or colleagues. Justice has many shades of interpretation unlike the other three because it may relate to rationing; an egalitarian approach to scarce resources or a sense of fairness in ensuring that care is given according to need alone.

14.2 **Certainty**

One of the most common confounding issues in ethical debates is the concept of certainty. Decisions and subsequent actions are usually easy when all the facts are known and there is a logical process to follow. Setting an anaesthetic ventilator is an example; the laws of physics will dictate the mechanical actions and performance of the gases involved. Precise measurements can be made to confirm that the desired effect has been achieved. Unfortunately clinical practice is nowhere near so clear-cut. We may have risk indices that predict a 90% mortality with an operation, but of the ten, which patient survives is impossible to predict. It is against such a lack of clarity that we use ethical processes in our daily practice.

We are all too frequently beset by the law of unintended consequences. We can debate with the patient the likely risks and benefits of a course of action but we cannot provide any guarantees. The deeper we go in to trying to describe the influences that may have an impact on the outcome, the more likely we are to confuse the patient. Making the judgement on how much to discuss, how much to explain and when to leave out the finer details varies with each patient.

14.3 **Consent**

In this context, consent means seeking a patient's agreement for the provision of care. It is a process that starts as soon as the patient is seen and continues to discharge from care. There are moments where a more formal process is invoked; signing a document agreeing to an operation for example, but the whole delivery of care to that patient involves consent.

Consent, to be valid, has to meet certain criteria. For example, the patient must be competent to make the decision, it has to be given without duress and it must be fully informed. It also serves at least three purposes: it provides a legal framework to defend against criminal charges such as assault, it recognizes the autonomy of the patient in determining their future and it should have a clear clinical purpose to make it necessary.

There are legal limitations on who can give consent, and, while these differ across the world, the European Convention on Human Rights enshrines those individual rights that are relevant to this aspect of medical law. These include the protection of the right to life, freedom of thought and the prohibition of torture, inhuman or degrading treatment or punishment among others. In the UK, consent can be given by the following:

- Adults over the age of 18
- Children over the age of 16
- 'Gillick' competent children under the age of 16

This differs from the ability to give consent in cases in which children who could give consent refuse to do so in which case this can be overruled by either a person with parental responsibility or the court if it is in their best interests.

14.4 **Voluntariness**

Decisions that the patient makes with regard to consent must be made without duress or under coercion. In the elderly, this may be difficult to ascertain because many frail elderly patients do not want to 'burden' their families and will try to choose options with their families' interests at heart rather than their own wishes. Many frail patients are vulnerable to pressure from other carers or even friends to accept or refuse treatment.

14.5 Information

There is a duty of care to provide as much information to the patient as to allow them to make an informed choice about their treatment options. This is not the same as the patient's right to know. Until recently a defence on how much information should be given was that that a 'responsible body of medical opinion' would have provided. However, it is now clear that there are several descriptions of risks that should be disclosed. These are risks that are
- Obviously necessary
  - This is a risk so obviously necessary that no reasonably prudent medical man would fail to disclose it. Dying during a ruptured aortic aneurysm repair for instance.
- Special risks
  - These are risks that are specific to that patient or in form or severity. Paralysis following odontoid surgery in the neck perhaps.
- Significant risks
  - These are risks that would affect the judgement of a reasonable patient. This research is likely to kill you but it is worth it!

The information being provided to the patient must be in a form and at a time that they can understand. It is worth keeping in mind that there is a high level of illiteracy in the UK population and this remains true in the elderly; estimates are of 5–10%. Frightened patients do not remember well, and most of the information given after the bad news is likely to be poorly recalled if at all. Repeating information and presenting it in different ways improve assimilation and understanding.

The elderly have significant communication problems as well. Almost 35% are very deaf and the same percentage is almost blind. The combination of the two, blindness and deafness, makes giving information (and signing the consent form) difficult. Pictures and diagrams are usually better than written material although patient information leaflets (see RCOA website) are very helpful sources that can be referred to again and again.

Suggested areas that should be given to all patients include the following:
- The reason for the consent.
- An explanation of the problem.

- What options there are for treatment, including doing nothing.
- What the surgery (if that is an option) entails.
- What the risks and complications are.
- Post-operative expectations – length of convalescence for instance.

These should be evidence based and regularly reviewed. They should have a 'review-by-date' and ideally be available in a range of locally used languages.

14.6 **Who should seek consent?**

It is the duty of care of the doctor providing treatment or ordering investigations to discuss the reasons with the patient and explain the risks involved. To do this the doctor must have a comprehensive understanding of both the procedure and their competence in it. Delegation should be rare, but if necessary it should be to another person who has been trained and assessed as competent to seek consent with appropriate knowledge of the procedure or investigation and the associated risks.

14.7 **Competence/capacity**

Capacity in this instance is the ability or power to do, experience or understand something. Patients have to be able to understand what is being said to them, believe that it is true and retain the information for long enough to consider it as part of making their decision. There are different levels of capacity relating to the decisions being taken.

Capacity does not equate to making a reasonable decision. Irrational decisions, if the consequences of that decision are understood, have to be accepted. The only person who can give consent apart from the patient is someone who has been nominated with lasting power of attorney (LPA) under the new Mental Capacity Act.

In the UK, the Mental Capacity Act 2005 (http://www.dca.gov.uk/capacity/index.htm) has enshrined case law into a statute to provide protection for those who lack capacity. This includes those with learning difficulties as well as the cognitively impaired elderly patient. The fundamental principle is that of autonomy and capacity has to be assumed to be present until proved otherwise. Equally, all reasonable steps have to be taken to assist the patient to understand. There are two stages to determining capacity under this act. The first asks whether there is a disturbance or impairment in cognition that could make them unable to make a decision. This dysfunction could be temporary, delirium or drug related, or it could be permanent, following a head injury or in severe dementia. The second relates to the decision process itself, with all the issues of understanding and retaining information as well as being able to decide and communicate that decision (Box 14.1).

129

> ## Box 14.1 Key principles of the Mental Capacity Act 2005
>
> - A person must be assumed to have capacity unless it is established that they lack capacity.
> - A person cannot be treated as unable to make a decision unless all practicable steps to help them do so have been taken without success.
> - A person cannot be treated as unable to make a decision merely because they make an unwise decision.
> - You must act, or make decisions, on behalf of a person who lacks capacity in their best interests.
> - Before you act or make a decision, you must consider whether the purpose for which it is needed can be as effectively achieved in a way that is less restrictive of the person's rights and freedom of action.

Other factors to consider will include such aspects as previously expressed wishes, the views of close relatives, their beliefs and so on. The relevant factors must not be restricted to medical issues.

The act creates a new advocate for the patient in that they can nominate an individual to have LPA. Only competent adults can nominate someone as an LPA, but it gives them rights not only over property and financial areas (which were in the previous provision) but also over decisions on health care and medical treatment. Withdrawal of treatment decisions can be implemented only if the patient while competent expressly documented them.

The creation of a new court of protection, the ability of the court to appoint deputies to act for patients lacking capacity and independent advocates for those who do not have others to speak for them are all provisions that will protect patients as well as the medical attendants.

14.8 Euthanasia

The right to life has been linked to the right to choose when to die since the early part of the last century. So far only a few countries have legalized this and there has been little progress in the UK. The risks inherent in providing care for vulnerable and frail elderly patients if this process became legal are great. They are especially at risk from close relatives or carers who seek financial return from their relative's death.

Unfortunately the right to the provision of a dignified, pain free death in a suitable pleasant environment has increasingly been tied to the right to choose when to die. The two are not the same; one is a demand for highly skilled palliative care teams for all who need them and the other is for a means to be legally killed when life becomes unbearable. Society, ultimately, will have to make their judgement on this issue although medicine will require that refusing to provide this will not be seen as a failure to provide a duty of care.

14.9 Summary

The ethical issues around consent and capacity are central to the care of the elderly patient and a clear understanding of the principles is necessary. There are recent changes in UK legislation that we need to be aware of as part of our daily practice and our own personal planning for the future.

Further reading

Guidance to healthcare professionals http://www.dca.gov.uk/legal-policy/mental-capacity/mibooklets/guide3.pdf.

The Mental Capacity Act 2005, http://www.dca.gov.uk/capacity/index.htm.

Index

N

O

P